How I Survived Prostate Cancer ...and So Can You

A Guide for Diagnosing and Treating Prostate Cancer

James Lewis, Jr., Ph.D.

How I Survived Prostate Cancer
...and So Can You

A Guide for Diagnosing and Treating Prostate Cancer

James Lewis, Jr., Ph.D.

HEALTH EDUCATION LITERARY PUBLISHER
An Affiliate of the NationalCenter to Save Our Schools
Westbury, New York

Published by Health Education Literary Publisher
P.O. Box 948
Westbury, New York 11590

Health Education Literary Publisher is an affiliate of the National Center to Save Our Schools

Permission to reprint two quotes from the book, *The Prostate Book*, by Stephen N. Rous, M.D., published by W.W. Norton & Company, N.Y., 1992, pp. 171-172 and p. 174.

Permission to reprint the incidence of prostate cancer chart from the book, *Prostate Problems: The Complete Guide to Their Treatment*, by Jeremy Hamand, published by Thorsons, an imprint of HarperCollins Publishers, Hammersmith, London, England, 1991, p. 130

Library of Congress Cataloging-in-Publication Data

Lewis, James, 1930-
How I survived prostate cancer—and so can you: a guide for
    diagnosing and treating prostate cancer/James Lewis,
    PI cm,
    Includes bibliographical references and index,
    ISBN 1-883257-06-9
    1, Prostate—Cancer—Popular works, I. Title.
    RC280.P7L49 1994
    616.99'463—dc2o   94-10168
                                            CIP

Manufactured in the United States of America

Dedication

This book is dedicated:

To all of my childhood friends who are not alive today because of the toll of poverty.

To all of my colleagues in the two prostate cancer support groups who stimulated my thinking and guided me in researching and writing this book.

To all of the physicians who reviewed and edited this book and those with whom I interacted and disagreed, thus helping me in my thought processes.

To all of the prostate cancer specialists in the world who are striving to prove that some nontraditional treatments for prostate cancer may be more effective and have less side effects than the traditional treatments.

Finally, to the memory of my mother, two brothers, sister, mother-in-law, and father-in-law who have passed on to the other side, I am still trying to make a difference and need their help to continue my purpose in life.

Table Of Contents

Qualifying Statement

All of the information, suggestions, and recommendations made in this book are not meant to be "medical prescriptions," nor do I claim to be a medical doctor. The advice is based on my experience, readings, research, studies, and interactions with prostate cancer patients and various cancer specialists. It is written with the understanding that the author and publisher are not rendering medical or other professional services. The author, medical advisors, and publisher shall have neither liability nor responsibility to any person or entity with respect to any loss, harm, or damage caused or alleged to be caused directly or indirectly by the information contained in this book.

I have tried to keep my comments nonbiased. In fact, the physicians who reviewed and edited this book indicated when I was biased and I rewrote the context in regard to their recommendations. More than 286 recommendations were cited by the four physicians and the one survivor who reviewed and edited the original manuscript. I believe that the book has been enhanced as a result of their professional advice. When you read this book, I challenge you to discuss the contents with your doctors. Go to their offices with book in hand with underlined sections you want clarified. When in doubt, seek one, two, or more professional opinions, and if you are still in doubt, do what one of my physicians asked of me, "use your instincts."

Acknowledgements

I would like to thank all of the people who helped me to make this book a reality. I particularly want to express my appreciation to all of the physicians and the one prostate cancer survivor who served on my medical advisory board. I owe thanks to E. Roy Berger, M.D., my oncologist and one of the members of the team that was instrumental in getting the Food and Drug Administration (FDA) to approve flutamide as an acceptable prescriptive hormone for treating prostate cancer. Even though he was extremely busy with his practice in Smithtown, New York, Dr. Berger did afford me the opportunity to meet with him on several occasions to discuss and clarify recommendations he made regarding the text. I found these two sessions informative in that they expanded my knowledge of prostate cancer.

I owe much to my "nephew," Llewellyn M. Hyacinthe, M.D., a urologist, who I watched grow up from a little, inquisitive child to become a physician who is on the path toward becoming a diplomate in his chosen endeavor. Even though his schedule was full, he allocated sufficient time to review my book and to offer his professional recommendations, requiring me to make needed adjustments to the book.

I am extremely grateful to my radiation oncologist, who painstakingly reviewed my book, even though he was in the midst of a move. He generously cited at least fifty recommendations to improve my book. His comments about the book in general were extremely favorable and they were appreciated.

I owe thanks to Lloyd J. Ney, executive director of Patient Advocates for Advanced Cancer Treatments (PAACT), the largest nonprofit prostate cancer research organization in the world. Without PAACT's publications and Ney's comments, I doubt if I could have completed this book. I owe so much to this person who was given only three months to live and is now reaching his tenth year of survival after prostate cancer. God truly has a purpose for him.

I owe thanks to my son, Michael J. Lewis, a registered certified physician assistant, who helped me with the research and to interpret the current medical terminology and procedures. Other members of my family who helped to collect research and articles on prostate cancer were my wife Valdmir, my other son Terence, and my daughter, Patricia Lewis Johnson.

I certainly cannot forget my administrative assistant, Lisa Bolognese, who painstakingly diagnosed my poor penmanship, corrected my spelling and at time grammar to help me to produce this book. I am grateful for her assistance.

I am also thankful to numerous other prostate cancer specialists whom I contacted for information, clarification, and recommendations. The learning journey I took to write this book would not have been possible had it not been for the hundreds of prostate cancer patients who educated me and for those whom I educated. I am convinced that without a doubt, everything this book is resulted in part from the personal relationships I had with my colleagues in the two prostate cancer support groups that I attend.

Finally, once again, I would like to thank all those who made this book and my growth possible. Now it is time for me to carry on and continue as an educator to influence others until my book of life is completed.

James Lewis, Jr., Ph.D.

Why I Wrote This Book

There is an old adage: "What you don't know won't hurt you." This is not true when you relate it to prostate cancer. Then, these words should be changed to, "what you don't know may kill you." That is why I wrote this book: To lengthen or to save your life! If you have prostate cancer, it is important for you to become an active learner, that is, to read, research, and talk to everybody who has an interest in prostate cancer. What was true yesterday may not be true today. A practice used yesterday may be obsolete today. For example, I was diagnosed with prostate cancer in 1992. Prior to writing this book, my choice of treatment, as well as that of my urologist, was combination hormonal therapy, followed by external beam radiation. Knowing what I have learned through researching and writing this book, which is several months after my treatment, my first choice of treatment would be an examination of my lymph nodes, three to six months of combination hormonal therapy to debulk and downstage my prostate gland to make it more manageable for cryosurgery, which would then be administered by the world's greatest specialist in this field.

In 1994, 200,000 men will be diagnosed with prostate cancer and approximately 38,000 of them will die of the disease. American men have the highest incidence of prostate cancer in the world. In fact, every fifteen minutes, a man will die of prostate cancer in this country. If you are a white male, the chance that you will get this disease is 1 out of 11. If you are an African-American male, your chances are 1 out of 8. The reason for this difference is not known. Some believe it is because African-American men have a higher level of testosterone than do white men. It really doesn't matter. If you have prostate cancer, you must do something about it right now, not later—later is too late.

According to the 1990 U.S. census, there are about 23.4 million American men between the ages of 50 and 75, the optional screening years for prostate cancer. Data from autopsies conducted by John T. Isaacs, M.D., a medical oncologist at Johns Hopkins (Maryland) University, revealed that approximately 11 million men in this country have some form of prostate cancer. Using the information supplied by John McNeal, M.D., a pathologist in the department of urology at Stanford (California) University, who suggests that one out of five cases of prostate cancer becomes clinically significant, I estimate that 2.2 million men in America have clinical evidence of prostate cancer and 650 thousand of these will eventually die of the disease within a 15-year period.

The reasons for this may be partly due to those of us who do not get an annual physical examination and our physicians who fail to perform the simple digital rectal examination and PSA blood test during the physical examination. Perhaps the overall cause of the high incidence of prostate cancer and the cause of death to those for whom is was fatal is due to our "abundance of ignorance" when it comes to our bodies.

I recently saw a television program about prostate cancer in which the moderator was interviewing men in New York City about the location of the prostate gland. Some signalled that the prostate was on the left side of their heart; others stated it was on the right side of their stomach; while some did not know and laughed. I laughed, too. I should not have, because it highlights the significance of one of our problems.

To some extent, I cannot blame these men. You see, I am an educator and I had little knowledge about my prostate until I was springboarded into action because of my doctor's pronouncement that I had prostate cancer.

In this book, I am going to take you through the journey I used to learn about the number one cancer killer in men 50 years of age and older. I will introduce you to several basic items you should know about your prostate, such as the size and texture of your prostate, your blood test level or prostate specific antigen (PSA), your Gleason score, the characteristics of your prostate, your stage, and the battery of tests used to determine if your disease has spread. Armed with this information, you will be able to converse with your doctors without that "abundance of ignorance" I mentioned previously.

Thanks to the generosity of Patient Advocates for Advanced Cancer Treatment (PAACT) and its members, I have been able to share with you numerous letters and brief case histories of patients like yourself who have been afflicted with prostate cancer. I have also included some letters from physicians.

I will discuss the various choices of treatment for prostate cancer in easy-to-understand language. I will explain traditional and nontraditional procedures and describe their side effects. As I discuss and explain diagnostic techniques and treatments, I will indicate my personal experience so you can profit from my "licks and bruises." You will be exposed to the research to substantiate the point being made. One chapter is devoted to questionable practices so you can determine for yourself what is right and wrong by further study and interaction with other doctors.

I have devised a "PSA Trend Chart" so you can track your PSA level each time you visit your doctor to get a blood test. This chart will enable you to keep a watchful eye on the progress of your disease so you can take appropriate action, if warranted. In addition, I have developed a "Prostate Cancer Report Card" so you can relate to your doctor in an intelligent manner by recording and discussing each step in diagnosing your condition. You can also use your report card to get a second, and even a third opinion.

To give you some idea as to what you are in for when your choice of treatment is either radical prostatectomy, external beam radiation, or a nontraditional treatment, I will explain what happens before, during, and after each one of these and other typical prostate cancer treatments.

Because support groups were a big help for me in gathering materials for my research and reading, and in interacting with doctors and any colleagues who were as thirsty for knowledge as I, I have also included resources for you to get support. For instance, sometimes a person comes along who will not accept death even though the doctor only gave him three to six months to live. He is what we call a champion and his weapon is flutamide when used in combination with luprolide. Using these hormone suppressors as a springboard, this champion, Lloyd Ney, founded PAACT. I will discuss the function of this organization as well as the other support groups that educated me.

Further, I will discuss combination hormonal therapy, which has saved or lengthened hundreds of thousands of lives throughout the world, even though professionals are still trying to determine its effectiveness. Throughout the manuscript, I include the opinions of the physicians who reviewed and edited this book, particularly when they disagreed with my research or the practice of one or more of my personal doctors.

I did not write this book solely for patients with prostate cancer, but also for the wives, children, relatives, and friends who want to improve their knowledge of the disease. In this way, all concerned individuals can determine for themselves what is the best way to support their loved one as he travels the journey to complete cure, remission, or a lengthened survival time.

Not only was I affected by the announcement by my doctor that I had prostate cancer, so were my wife, children, relatives, and friends. I will explain their concerns and what I did to accommodate them, down to preparing a living will. Because I feel it is important for you to select the best doctor possible to diagnose and treat your prostate cancer, I will give you some tips as to how I did it. By the way, I also did some things wrong. I will cite these, and explain what I would have done differently.

Finally, when all traditional and nontraditional treatments fail, I will discuss other options to perhaps prolong or save your life. I also devote some attention to what your options are should you have a recurrence of prostate cancer. Further, for your easy reference, I begin my book by citing the "Ten Commandments" for diagnosing and treating prostate cancer.

I hope that my experiences and those of other men with prostate cancer who are cited in this book will be helpful in giving you not only physical, but also psychological comfort as you journey down the road for a cure or proper treatment for your disease. Hold onto this guide, and from time to time refer to it to refresh your memory and to guide your actions.

James Lewis, Jr., Ph.D.

April 1994

PREFACE

I have been a student of prostate cancer for more than ten years. The more I learn, the more questions I have. As a medical oncologist who first became interested in this disease through clinical trials done in collaboration with Dr. Fernand Labrie in Quebec, Canada, I have tried to look at the multitude of diagnostic and therapeutic options objectively. This has not been an easy task as there are still much data to be gathered and interpretations to be made. The field is in a great state of flux. As an example of the confusion that currently reigns: I recently attended a meeting of physicians who have a special interest in treating prostate cancer. The moderator, a well-known academic urologist, said he wanted to hear how the members of the audience, mostly urologists with a smattering of medical oncologists, radiation therapists, and endocrinologists, would treat these patients. He prefaced the presentation with a statement that had a lasting impact on me. He said there weren't necessarily any right or wrong answers. I knew we did not know a lot about prostate cancer, but I did not think our knowledge was quite that primitive. As the seminar proceeded, case after case was presented. Rarely was there any consensus from the group on the optimal way to treat almost every case presented. The point I am trying to make is: If the physicians who treat this disease on a regular basis cannot agree on a treatment most of the time, can a patient make any sensible choice when faced with this difficult therapeutic dilemma, especially when his life hangs in the balance?

James Lewis, Jr., Ph.D. has been my patient for the past two years. Being an educator, his mission has been and remains to impart knowledge to his fellow man. This book is the culmination of Dr. Lewis' quest for and attainment of a great deal of knowledge about prostatic cancer. It was obtained out of the necessity of understanding what his choices were. I personally have spent a lot of time with him explaining the current state of knowledge in the field, mostly as it relates to his particular case, but as an editor we delved into diagnosis, pathologic grade and scoring, staging and therapeutic options. He did a great deal of research on his own and has reached certain biases, conclusions, and recommendations in which he strongly believes.

A lot of what Dr. Lewis recommends has scientific basis albeit some of the data is perhaps too early for the medical community to condone as the current recommended therapy. I, however, as already mentioned, rarely have seen a group of prostate cancer specialists agree on one simple way to treat this disease.

This book is an attempt to demystify the different options a prostate cancer patients faces today. If nothing else, it will open the patient's eyes to those options. The individual with his physician(s) must choose the best course for himself. This is where the art and science of medicine interact. What is good medicine for one patient may be absolutely anathema to another. In choosing a course of action, many variables need to be taken into account. These include not only the medical, but also the psychosocial and sexual repercussions of the various treatment modalities including observation only. Until the patient and his family truly understand what the various options are and the consequences these may have, a truly informed decision cannot be reached.

I expect this work to engender a fair amount of criticism from healthcare professionals who either are indoctrinated in their own bias systems or accuse Dr. Lewis of operating on his own set of dogma. Only time and more clinical trials will tell who is correct.

This book will hopefully alert patients and their families to the options available. Research is continuously ongoing and as more information is collected, treatment options may change. I expect many sequels of this book or ones like it to be necessary to keep the public up-to-date on the state of the art on diagnosis and treatment of prostate cancer.

E. Roy Berger, M.D.
Medical Oncologist

The Ten Commandments For Diagnosing And Treating Prostate Cancer

1. THOU SHALL GET AN ANNUAL PHYSICAL EXAMINATION CONSISTING OF A DIGITAL RECTAL EXAMINATION AND A PROSTATE SPECIFIC ANTIGEN (PSA) BLOOD TEST IF THEE IS FORTY YEARS OF AGE OR OLDER.

2. THOU SHALL INSIST THAT A MINIMUM OF SIX PUNC-TURES BE PERFORMED WHEN UNDERGOING A BIOPSY UNDER THE GUIDANCE OF A TRANSRECTAL ULTRA-SOUND MACHINE IF AN ELEVATED PSA LEVEL IS DETER-MINED AFTER A REPEATED TEST.

3. THOU SHALL KNOW THE SIZE AND TEXTURE OF THEE PROSTATE GLAND, PSA LEVEL, GLEASON SCORE, STAGE, CHARACTERISTICS OF THY CANCER CELLS, AND RESULTS OF VARIOUS TESTS AND USE SAME FOR ASSISTING THEE PHYSICIAN IN ARRIVING AT A MUTUAL CHOICE OF TREATMENT.

4. THOU SHALL REQUEST TO BE PUT ON COMBINATION HORMONAL THERAPY FOR SIX MONTHS AS A PRELIMI-NARY TREATMENT FOR MOST STAGES OF THEE DISEASE.

5. THOU SHALL GET A SECOND AND EVEN A THIRD PROFES-SIONAL OPINION ONCE THEE HAS BEEN DIAGNOSED AND A TREATMENT HAS BEEN RECOMMENDED BY A PHYSI-CIAN.

6.   THOU SHALL RESEARCH AND STUDY THE LITERATURE ON PROSTATE CANCER, INTERACT WITH OTHERS, AND JOIN AT LEAST ONE PROSTATE CANCER SUPPORT GROUP IN ORDER TO FORTIFY THYSELF WITH INFORMATION IN AN EFFORT TO INTELLIGENTLY INTERACT WITH THEE PHYSICIAN.

7.   THOU SHALL INTEGRATE PHYSICAL HEALING WITH DIETARY AND PSYCHOLOGICAL HEALINGS TO CONQUER PROSTATE CANCER ON ALL FRONTS.

8.   THOU SHALL BE AS SENSITIVE IN SELECTING A TREATMENT FOR PROSTATE CANCER AND THE MEDICAL TECHNOLOGY FOR THE ADMINISTRATION OF THE TREATMENT AS THEE ARE IN SELECTING A PHYSICIAN.

9.   THOU SHALL ACT IMMEDIATELY TO UNDERGO ADDITIONAL TESTS REQUESTED BY THE PHYSICIAN SUCH AS LYMPH NODES ANALYSIS, CT SCAN, BONE SCAN, X-RAY, MRI, AND ANY OTHER TESTS TO COMPLETE THY DIAGNOSTIC STUDY.

10. THOU SHALL MONITOR THEE PSA LEVEL ONCE A TREATMENT HAS BEEN PERFORMED FOR A PERIOD OF THREE MONTHS AFTER TREATMENT AND EVERY SIX AND/OR TWELVE MONTHS THEREAFTER TO DETERMINE IF THERE IS A STEADY RISE IN THE PSA LEVEL IN AN EFFORT TO BE ALERT TO A RECURRENCE OF PROSTATE CANCER.

CHAPTER ONE

What I Learned and What You Should Know About Prostate Cancer

I have prostate cancer. Why, I don't know. Twelve years ago, I had colon cancer. Some physicians say there is and some say there is not a correlation between colon cancer and prostate cancer. Numerous studies suggest that it may be due to my diet, consisting sometimes of red meats, dairy and white flour products, and foods rich in sugar, which over time can accumulate and turn into tumors. However, I have not found any definitive study to once and for all settle this matter, even though a new study from the Harvard School of Public Health indicated that men who ate red meat five or more times per week were 2.5 times more likely to suffer from advanced prostate cancer than men who ate red meat once a week or less. Some scientists say that toxic chemicals and electromagnetic fields are possible causes of cancer; however, I have not been involved in any recent wars or been exposed to any toxic chemicals, nor do I live near any electromagnetic fields.

A few studies indicate that prostate cancer patients consume less foods that contain certain vitamins, but I know of a number of friends and colleagues who take from six to fifteen vitamins, including zinc daily and some of them have prostate cancer. Some studies mention that heredity is a strong factor for developing prostate cancer. Although my father is ninety-four years old, his doctor says he has no signs of prostate cancer. A study done in Iceland revealed that there may be an increased risk of prostate cancer in men whose mothers have had breast cancer. I do not know if my mother had breast cancer; however, I do know that when she died at the age of sixty-seven, she had nodules throughout her body.

True, I had an enlarged prostate prior to being diagnosed with prostate cancer, but some 400,000 men each year have an enlarged prostate, and many of them do not have prostate cancer. The literature suggests that there is no relationship between benign prostate hyperplasia (enlarged prostate) and prostate cancer, although many men with prostate cancer also have enlarged prostates.

One researcher reports that the average age of men who are diagnosed as having prostate cancer is 70. However, I was 61 when I was diagnosed with prostate cancer. Research seems to indicate that men in the U.S. have the highest incidence of prostate cancer in the world, particularly African-American men. In fact, the 1990 United States census indicates that there are approximately 4 million African-American men between the ages of 40 and 75. Using the data from both Drs. John T. Isaacs and John McNeal (both mentioned in the introduction) and the fact that the rate of prostate cancer among African-American men is 37 percent higher than among white men, approximately 1.9 million African-American men will have some form of prostate cancer and over 500,000 will have clinical evidence of this disease. Apparently I am part of this group and hope that I will not be among the nearly 170,000 of these men who will eventually die of this disease.

The problem with prostate cancer is that we really do not know what causes it. If I am allowed to speculate, I believe that there is no one reason for prostate cancer, but rather a multitude of causative factors. In addition, we have not yet determined the best treatment for prostate cancer, even with the "gold standard" treatments. In this book, I will take you on a learning journey so you will be able to make the best decision possible, hopefully with your physician's assistance, to diagnose and treat your prostate cancer condition.

Your first concern if you have been told by your doctor that you have prostate cancer should be to learn as much about the disease as you can so you may intelligently reach accord with your doctor to determine proper treatment for your disease. One of the first steps I took was to join a prostate cancer support group.

At one of my prostate support group meetings, several new members were asked to inform the group where they were in terms of either diagnosing or treating their prostate cancer. One man who was only fifty years old, which is young to be stricken with prostate cancer, indicated that he is recovering from a radical prostatectomy (my words, not his). Each of the regular members of the group began to query him about his treatment. He was asked his prostate specific antigen (PSA) level, Gleason score, and stage. He responded, "I don't know what you are talking about. My doctor never informed me of these things." I immediately said, "You mean you let the doctor operate on you without knowing why?" His reply was, "He frightened me and said that if I didn't get an operation, I was risking my life."

Members of the group looked at each other and shook their heads in disbelief that the patient would let the doctor operate on him without having adequate knowledge about his disease, and disbelief that a professionally trained doctor would fail to properly communicate to his patient, contrary to the Hippocratic oath, and would frighten his patient into getting an operation.

Another member of the group said he did not know what we were talking about. He said these terms were new to him also, and that his doctor told him he had better see his lawyer and make out a will prior to his next appointment. We asked him what he did. He responded, "I cried."

We queried another new member of the support group and he said he was scheduled to receive seed implantation, but cancelled it because he felt that his doctor failed to give him enough information so he could feel comfortable with the decision. This new member said he felt insulted when he received the following letter from his doctor:

C.M., Brooklyn, N.Y.:

> It was brought to my attention that you have cancelled your Iodine-125 seed implantation of the prostate. I would like to advise you that I do not feel this is a wise decision. At this point in time your prostatic cancer is localized in the prostate. It is a Gleason 4, which means that it is a moderately actively growing tumor and the best time to treat this and have a long-term survival is when it is localized to the prostate. Your past history of hypertension as well as having TURP in 1987, [sic] the best form of treatment at this point in time would be a combination radiotherapy consisting of seed implantation of the prostate followed by external beam radiation.

It is interesting to denote that a Gleason score of 4 is a well-differentiated cancer and not a moderately differentiated cancer, as stated by the doctor. (A Gleason score identifies the aggressiveness of the cancer. I will discuss this later in the chapter.) Further discussion revealed that our new colleague never received an explanation as to all of the treatment options available to him and the advantages and disadvantages of each one.

These three stories were not new to the veteran members of the prostate cancer support group. Because I attend two support groups, I have listened to numerous stories in which men with prostate cancer were told little about their disease and relied solely on their doctor to determine their fate. I promised that if and when I wrote a book about prostate cancer, the first chapter would discuss essential information all men should know about the disease so they will be able to join their doctors in arriving at a mutually agreed upon treatment plan. After all, no one has a greater stake in arriving at a decision in the determination of his fate than the person who has been diagnosed with prostate cancer.

Figure 1.1
Portions of the Male Reproductive System

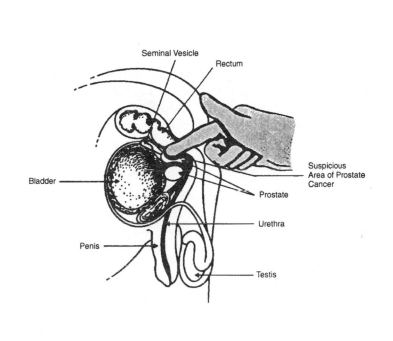

WHAT IS THE PROSTATE?

Your prostate gland is often referred to as an accessory sex gland. This is because even though its sole purpose is sexual, it is only indirectly involved in procreation. The prostate gland is located below the bladder and in front of your rectum, as illustrated in Figure 1.1. It is the size of a walnut and reddish brown in color. The purpose of the gland is to produce semen, the grayish heavy fluid that occurs during ejaculation and carries sperm from the testicles. Your prostate gland needs the male sex hormone, testosterone to function properly. Testosterone is produced by the testicles. However, the adrenal gland also produces a small amount of male sex hormone. This is an important point to remember for future reference. The average size of the prostate gland is 20 grams. The size of the prostate gland is important because enlargement may indicate your difficulty. An enlarged prostate gland could indicate either benign prostate hyperplasia (BPH) or cancer of the prostate.

BPH is not a cancerous condition, and therefore does not spread to other parts of the body. It is more like a nuisance disease. The prostate gland becomes enlarged and pushes against the urethra and bladder, making urination somewhat difficult. The National Institutes of Health reports that half of the male population in the United States between the ages of sixty and seventy will acquire some degree of BPH. Usually an operation called transurectal prostate surgery, or TURP, is done to relieve a person with BPH. Now a pill called Proscar can be prescribed by your doctor to relieve you of the discomfort of BPH. However, Proscar does not work for everyone. There is another drug that works like Proscar. Serenoa repens is derived from the extract of the saw palmetto plant and comes in a preparation called permixon, which can be found in most health food stores.

PROSTATE CANCER

Cancer of the prostate is a very serious disease that must be given immediate attention. Cancer is a disease in which certain cells in the body have formed a malignant tumor that can invade and destroy healthy cells and tissues throughout your body, such as your lymph nodes, bones, liver, bladder, rectum, and other organs. When cancer of the prostate spreads to other parts of the body, it is known as metastatic prostate cancer.

During the early stages, prostate cancer may not show any symptoms whatsoever or may show nonspecific symptoms. Some of the symptoms that may signal cancer of the prostate are:

- Frequent urination
- Difficulty in either starting or holding the urine

- Inability to urinate

- Painful or burning urination

- Painful ejaculation

- Blood in the urine or semen

- Frequent pain in the lower back, hips, or upper thighs which may mean that prostate cancer has metastasized

- Swollen lymph glands

When you do experience any of the above symptoms, you must seek the immediate attention of a doctor, and request that he or she give you a complete medical examination. The sooner you accomplish this, the better.

Take my case, for example. At one time, I had five of the eight symptoms listed above, and was not diagnosed with cancer of the prostate. When my doctor told me that I had prostate cancer—and after I recovered from the revelation—all sorts of questions went through my mind. These included: How long would I have to live? Why was this happening to me? Why do I have cancer again? How will my family feel when I inform them? Can I continue my profession? How should I pursue treatment of my condition? Did my previous doctors miss something they should not have, which caused a delay in my diagnosis?, etc.

Of course, I went berserk with numerous questions. Once I settled down, I began to become more rational and analytical. I knew I had to learn more about diagnosis and treatment of prostate cancer so I could participate with my doctors, make informed decisions, and hopefully, ensure a long life for myself. I realized that I had to be careful in selecting doctors for a second, third, and even a fourth opinion. I knew that I had to involve my wife because of the impact the disease will have on her and our children. I knew that I had to talk to others who were either undergoing or completing their treatment. I knew that I had to join one or two support groups to learn from other men's experiences. I knew I had to make contact with various organizations to get information on the latest treatments. I knew what I had to do, and I had to do it immediately!

My investigation of the literature and my interaction with my doctors and colleagues convinced me that the first thing I had to comprehend was the several methods doctors use to diagnose prostate cancer. Doctors will or should examine the following:

1. The volume, size, and texture of your prostate gland;
2. The PSA level, which is a blood test;
3. The Gleason scoring or the aggressiveness of your prostate cancer;
4. The stage of advancement of your disease;
5. A DNA ploidy analysis, which characterizes the nature of your prostate cancer cells; and,
6. A battery of tests to determine if your prostate cancer has spread.

Each of these methods will be discussed in this chapter.

Ask Your Doctor How Your Prostate Cancer Feels

The first method your doctor will use to examine the condition of your prostate gland is the digital rectal examination. To do this, the doctor will insert his or her gloved finger into your rectum and feel your prostate for enlargement, stiffness, hardness, and nodules. This method usually takes about 30 seconds and may cause some discomfort. However, it should not be painful. Even though your entire prostate gland cannot be examined using the digital rectal method, your doctor can detect any unusual growths on the prostate where a tumor is likely to occur.

The average size of the prostate gland is reported to be at the weight of 60 grams. One of my doctors reported that my prostate was 80 grams, which is very large; however, the presence of prostate cancer is independent of the size of the gland.

Keep in mind that the digital rectal examination has a serious limitation. Research seems to report that less than 20 percent of prostate cancer can be detected using this method. In fact, it is reported that of those examined, the digital rectal examination misses nearly half of the early cases of prostate cancer, especially cancer growth, that is located in the front part of the gland, where the doctor's finger cannot touch. However, when the digital rectal examination is used with the prostatic specific antigen or PSA blood test, the detection rate for prostate cancer increases significantly to over 60 percent.

Another limitation of the digital rectal examination is when doctors forecast the stage of the disease. In a review of the literature by Glenn S. Gerber, M.D. and Gerald W. Chodak, M.D. it was found that up to 50 percent of tumors thought to be localized by digital rectal examination, i.e., Stage B, were subsequently upstaged on pathological staging to Stage D or D1 disease. In Thompson's survey, in which 17 patients were identified, 15 of whom were thought to have their disease confined to the prostate, 66 percent were upstaged. Therefore, of all prostate cancers diagnosed by digital rectal examination, only 30 to 40 percent were confined to the gland.

Another significant problem with the digital rectal examination is the infrequency with which is it performed on patients by both male and female doctors. In a screening program of 433 men over age 40, performed at the Cleveland Clinic in 1989 and 1990, 67 percent of the men said they did not have a digital rectal examination performed during the previous year. Even more alarming is the fact that of the 153 who reported having a general physical examination in the previous year, a digital rectal examination was performed on only 56 percent of the patients.

Before I began using my previous internist (who is now retired), I went to a female doctor for my annual examinations. However, not once in four years did she examine my prostate. If she continues this practice of avoidance, think of how many men she may adversely affect in her practice. Other colleagues of mine have echoed the same thing. Figure 1.2 illustrates the

and Texture of Prostate Gland

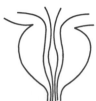

Normal prostate

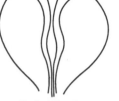

Benign prostatic
hypertrophy

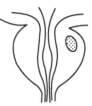

Early cancer
without a nodule;
tumor too small
to be detected
by rectal exam

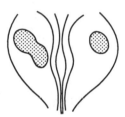

Early cancer with
enlarged prostate;
one or more nodules
confined to the
prostate; tumor large
enough to be detected
by rectal exam

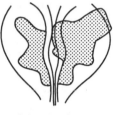

Enlarged prostate;
tumor has spread
beyond the capsule
often blocking the
urethra; can be
detected by rectal
exam

Enlarged prostate;
tumor has spread to
pelvic lymph nodes
and possibly to bones
and organs

various sizes and types of growths that can occur with the prostate gland. Reading from left to right, the first illustration shows the normal size of the prostate gland when compared with four enlarged prostates. The second illustration shows an enlarged benign prostate. The third illustration shows the normal size of the prostate with early signs of cancer on the right side. The fourth illustration shows an enlarged prostate with early signs of cancer on the left and right side. The fifth illustration shows an enlarged prostate with cancer outside the capsule. The final illustration shows an enlarged prostate with cancer that has spread throughout the body. An effective method to use to determine which one of these illustrations show the size and growth of your prostate is to show this figure to your doctor and ask him or her to select the one that best represents your condition.

Recommendation: Demand that your doctor conduct a digital rectal examination on you annually. If he or she has to be asked to do so, I would seriously consider seeking the attention of another doctor. When the digital rectal examination has been completed, ask your doctor if he or she feels any nodules or if your prostate feels normal or enlarged, hard, stiff, or lumpy. The desired condition is a prostate that feels normal in size and is smooth.

Know Your PSA Level

Even though your prostate gland may feel normal and smooth, the second method your doctor should use to diagnose your condition is to take a sample of your blood in order to get your prostate specific antigen or PSA level. The blood test detects a higher than normal level of protein that seeps out of the prostate gland when there is an abnormality. While reports indicate variations in terms of the detection rate of the PSA blood test, for prostate cancer the range seems to be from 53 to 70 percent, when used in conjunction with the digital rectal examination.

A study by the National Institute on Aging and Johns Hopkins University found that PSA levels usually begin rising 7 to 9 years before clinical diagnosis is made. This study found that PSA tests can detect 20 to 25 percent of prostate cancers an average of 4 years before diagnosis would be made without such tests. Another key finding is that repeat tests of measuring PSA levels over time significantly reduces the number of false negative readings, and thus leads to fewer unnecessary biopsies.

In 1988, when I had my first PSA blood test, it measured 13 nanograms per milliliter (ng/ml); the second test measured 15 ng/ml. Usually, if the first blood test indicates an elevated PSA level, the doctor then requests another blood test within 3 to 6 months to verify the previous test. Unfortunately, even though my first doctor was reported to be one of the best in the country, his associate failed to fully explain the significance of an elevated PSA level. I since have switched to one who is more sensitive to me as a person. My recommendation is that you read everything you can get your hands on to fully explain the meaning behind an elevated PSA level. Do not be afraid to ask your doctor questions about your PSA level and if necessary, challenge him or her with the knowledge you have attained from your readings.

Previously I mentioned some statistics in terms of physicians failing to give their patients an annual physical examination, which included a digital rectal examination and PSA blood test. However, physicians are not solely to blame; patients must also take the responsibility. The following have been cited as some of the reasons why men in America fail to get a physical examination for prostate cancer:

- Since in the early stage of prostate cancer there are usually no symptoms, men feel there is no need to get a physical examination.
- Many men feel it is not the "macho" thing to do.
- Many men do not like the idea of a doctor probing their rectum.
- Many men lack education concerning the seriousness of prostate cancer and the consequences if it is not detected early.
- Many men have a lack of access to facilities or funds for diagnosing and treating prostate cancer.
- Many men are afraid of facing a diagnosis of cancer, especially of a sexually-related gland.

Recently, I had an opportunity to participate on a panel with two urologists and a survivor of prostate cancer at the North General Hospital in Harlem, New York. Although hundreds of circulars were distributed throughout the community, only four men showed up for the panel. When I was asked how to solve the problem of a lack of interest, I replied, "Go out to churches and talk with congregations about prostate cancer. Tell them that over two million American men have prostate cancer. Tell them that nearly half of these men are walking around with prostate cancer about to or presently spreading throughout their bodies. Tell them about the fact that over one-half million of these men will eventually die of the disease. Tell them how painful it is to die of prostate cancer, even with our current therapies and medication. Tell them that prostate cancer can be cured if detected early."

I then switched my delivery, and said, "If that does not work, lay down the law. Say to your husbands or partners: 'No examination, no copulation [sex].'"

After the laughter quieted down, I told the group that I was serious and that wives can play an integral role in getting their husbands to the doctor for a physical examination. I suggest using one or more of the following methods:

1. Schedule an appointment for your spouse and go with him to the doctor. Speak to the doctor and make certain he or she performs a digital rectal examination and takes a PSA blood test. Follow the blood test with a telephone call to determine his PSA level and record it on the PSA trend chart.
2. Keep reminding him to get a physical examination until you become a nuisance. Keep at it until he goes for the physical examination.
3. Get your children involved and have them encourage their father to go for a physical examination and report the results to the whole family.
4. Call the doctor clandestinely and have him or her send an overnight express mail letter to your husband stating that it is important for him to see the doctor immediately. Do not let on that you contacted the doctor.

5. Make an appointment with your family doctor and have your husband go along with you. Request your doctor to examine him also.
6. Mutually agree on a date for both of you to go to the doctor for a physical examination.
7. Arrange to have your doctor come to the house to conduct the physical examination, although in some areas of the country, this may not be possible. The physicians may desire additional compensation for this service.
8. Request the priest, minister, or rabbi to convey to the congregation how important it is for their male parishioners to get an annual physical examination and to actually ask the men for their PSA levels.
9. Bribe your spouse by insisting that he get a physical examination, or you will no longer cook until he does; when he does, cook him his favorite meal.
10. Be silent and do not speak to your husband until he gets a physical examination, and when he does, have the family give him an award.
11. Use scare tactics. Describe in vivid detail the terrible pain associated with advanced stage prostate cancer.

Despite the seeming exaggerated tactics above, of which I am quite serious, since the advent of the PSA blood test, more and more men have been diagnosed with prostate cancer. This does not mean that the PSA level is an accurate assessment of a person with cancer of the prostate. It does mean there is an abnormality of the prostate gland. Anything above 4.0 ng/ml using the Hybritech test is a signal for further study. If your physician uses the Ablin test, there will be a different range of normalcy. One of the things I have to caution you about is if a subsequent biopsy does not show any indication of cancer, do not think you are free of the disease. The prostate cancer could be so minute that the biopsy missed the points of development, and it may be only a matter of time before a more accurate diagnosis is made about your disease. This is what happened to me. My first biopsy failed to reveal prostate cancer after an elevated PSA level of 13.0 ng/ml. To this day, I believe that my doctor was at fault for not detecting it earlier. I was used as a "guinea pig" so the doctors in the office could learn how to use the newly purchased ultrasound technology. The salesman was making professional decisions as to where the probe should be directed and where punctures should be made, and as a result, I only received two punctures. Several months ago, I asked three urologists about the minimum number of punctures a person should receive during a biopsy of the prostate. One urologist explained that he would have punctured me at least a half dozen times and if nothing was found, he would have requested that I come back in three months for a follow-up. Another experienced urologist in New York City, to whom I went for a third opinion, stated that he would have put me in the hospital and conducted about nine punctures to locate any abnormalities. My regular urologist punctured me about eight times in areas of suspicion. He located the cancer in two areas at an elevated PSA level of 41.0 ng/ml.

Recommendation: When undergoing a biopsy of the prostate, have your doctor report to you and make certain a minimum of six punctures are made.

A colleague I met at my college reunion was recovering from a TURP and had an elevated PSA of 768.0 ng/ml, but was not diagnosed with cancer. I understand that a TURP operation usually elevates a man's PSA level. My regular urologist indicated that he has a patient who has had an elevated PSA in the area of 700 for 8 years and he has not found any traces of cancer of the prostate.

Research seems to indicate that when the PSA level rises by 0.75 ng/ml in one year, cancer of the prostate may be indicated (technically, this phenomenon is known as PSA velocity), however, this data has recently been challenged. All of my reviewers maintain that it is more important to watch for an upward trend in your PSA level. Another method to determine the presence of cancer is to determine the size of the prostate by an ultrasound probe placed into the rectum. The smaller

Figure 1.3
PSA Trend Chart

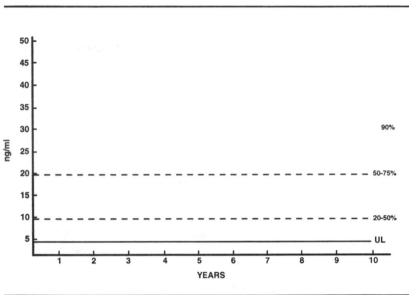

the size of the prostate, the greater the probability that a moderately elevated PSA is a sign of prostate cancer.

One method I used to track my PSA was the use of a PSA trend chart as illustrated in Figure 1.3. Every time I went to my physician and received a PSA blood test, I asked for my PSA level. Later, when I returned home, I charted the date and my PSA level with a dot, connecting it with the previous dot level. The first horizontal line represents the upper limits of the PSA level, meaning that when your PSA level reaches around 4.0 ng/ml, further diagnostic study is warranted. The first broken horizontal line represents a 20 to 50 percent probability of cancer, and the second broken line represents a 50 to 75 percent probability of prostate cancer. Anything above 20.04 ng/ml may indicate a 90 percent probability of prostate cancer. However, it must be realized that an elevated PSA only means that an abnormal condition exists. The following are potential reasons for elevated PSA levels: prostatitis, or infection of the prostate; benign prostate enlargement; and transurectal resection, or TURP for short.

Some interesting facts about the prostate and PSA levels are as follows:

- When prostate cancer has been removed through a radical prostatectomy, the PSA level should drop off to nearly zero. If it does not, there is a high probability that prostate tissue or cancer has been left in you.

- The PSA test can detect cancer of the prostate before you notice any symptoms; however, it may locate cancers that might not cause you any harm if left unattended.

- If after six months of radiation therapy your PSA level has not gone below the 4.0 ng/ml level, there is a high probability that cancer still exists in the prostate gland.

- Prostate cancer can exist with a normal PSA level.

- Prostate cancer may not exist with a high PSA level.

- Sometimes the test fails to detect a tumor.

- At times, the test appears to find a tumor where none actually exists.

- Several factors can temporarily inflate a PSA reading, such as BPH, prostatitis, or transurectal resection of the prostate. On the other hand, Proscar, a drug used to counteract BPH, can reduce the readings on the PSA test.

- The best way to use PSA readings is to continually track each of your PSA readings on the PSA trend chart.

- A continual rise in PSA level after treatment may indicate a recurrence of prostate cancer.

- Approximately one out of four men with a PSA of between 3.0 ng/ml and 4.0 ng/ml will have prostate cancer.

Critical PSA Levels and Recommended Actions

I am not a medical doctor, however, I have taken it upon myself to suggest certain critical PSA levels that should trigger

Figure 1.4
Critical PSA Levels and Recommended Action

Critical PSA Levels	Recommendations
PSA level between 0 and 4.0 ng/ml	Using the Hybritech/Abbott method, consider these values as normal. However, do not rely solely on the PSA level since some patients with localized prostate cancer have normal PSA level
PSA level between 3.0 and 4.0 ng/ml	Research seems to suggest that 25% of men with a PSA at this level will have prostate cancer in its early stage. Visit your physician every six months to monitor your PSA level
PSA level between 4.1 and 6.0 ng/ml	If you have not been diagnosed with prostate cancer and your PSA is at this level, you should return to your physician's office in three to six months and receive another PSA blood test. If a biopsy confirms that you have prostate cancer, you may be an appropriate patient for watchful waiting, that is, do nothing but monitor your disease, providing you are 70 years of age or older, have ten years or more to live, are in good health, your Gleason score is 4.0 ng/ml or less, you have been staged A or B, and your prostate cancer cells have been characterized as diploid.
PSA level between 6.1 and 10.0 ng/ml	This mild elevated PSA level does not necessarily mean you have prostate cancer. You may have prostatis which can be treated with antibodies, or BPH which can be treated with either surgery or medication. Your PSA level should be rechecked and if two ailments cited above are ruled out and your PSA level remains about the same, your physicians should give you a transrectal ultrasound examination followed by a biopsy.
PSA level above 10.0 ng/ml	Prostate cancer is more likely. Request your physician to recheck your PSA level and if it remains beyond this level, ask him or her to give you a biopsy guided by a transredtal ultrasound machine followed with several other tests, such as a CT scan, etc. Get to know your Gleason score, stage, and the characteristics of your prostate cancer cells.
PSA level above 20.0 ng/ml	Your physician should determine the extent of your prostate cancer and request analysis of your seminal vesicles and lymph nodes by using a rectal coil MRI using an imaging agent. However, one of my physicians questions the accuracy of this test. Prior to radical prostatectomy, seed implantation, or other treatments, the rest of your lymph nodes may need to be analzed via laparoscopy

some action on the part of your physician and yourself. These critical PSA levels and recommended actions as illustrated in Figure 1.4 are only guidelines and are not "carved in stone."

Once the digital rectal examination and PSA blood test reveal the need for additional study, the doctor should call you in for a biopsy guided by a transrectal ultrasound machine. By viewing the screen, your doctor can see nodules, calcium deposits, and other suspicious areas. At each suspicious site, he will insert a needle and collect a specimen. Usually, your doctor will insert the needle six to nine times to cover all the suspicious areas. Do not let your physician perform a biopsy on you unless he or she uses a transrectal ultrasound machine. However, my reviewers informed me that sometimes a clear and firm nodule can be easily biopsied without the use of an ultrasound machine. Until now, the punctures made by your physician when performing a biopsy were somewhat painful. In fact, since pain is relative, some men complained of sweating profusely during the process. It seems as though the more punctures were performed, the more pain was felt. I call this the accumulative pain phenomenon because the intensity of the puncture stayed the same and did not increase, it only felt that way because of the number of punctures. Currently, a new plastic biopsy device with a pistol grip shape makes it easier to diagnose prostate cancer, and since the needle is smaller than with other procedures, any pain is diminished.

Be Sure to Ask Your Doctor About the Stage of Your Cancer

Your chance of recovery (your prognosis) and choice of treatment depend on the stage of your cancer (whether it is just in the prostate or has spread to other parts of the body) and your general state of health. Once cancer of the prostate has been found (diagnosed), more tests will be done to find out if cancer cells have spread from the prostate to tissues around it or to other parts of the body. This is called staging. Your doctor needs to know the stage of your disease to help determine your treatment.

The following is a modified clinical staging system. If we were to use the modern TNM staging system, the stages would be different.

STAGE A: Prostate cancer at this stage cannot be felt and causes no symptoms. The cancer is only in the prostate and usually is found accidentally when surgery is done for other reasons, such as for BPH.

Stage A1: Well-differentiated tumor is found in one, two, or three areas of the prostate or less than 5 percent of the volume of tissue removed. (See page 22.)

Stage A2: Well-differentiated tumor is found in more than three areas of the prostate or any quantity of poorly differentiated tumor or more than 5 percent of the volume of tissue removed.

STAGE B: The tumor can be felt in the prostate during a rectal exam, but the cancer cells are found only in the prostate gland.

Stage B1: The tumor is confined to the prostate and usually can be felt during a rectal examination of the prostate. It is less than 1.5 centimeters in diameter, involves less than one lobe, and is surrounded on three sides by normal prostate.

Stage B2: The tumor is confined to the prostate, usually can be felt during a rectal examination of the prostate, is 1.5 centimeters or more in diameter, or involves a whole lobe, both lobes, or bilateral nodules.

Stage B3: The tumor is confined to the prostate, usually can be felt during a rectal examination of the prostate, and one tumor involves both lobes or nodules in both lobes.

STAGE C: Cancer cells have spread outside the covering (capsule) of the prostate to tissues around the prostate. The glands that produce semen (the seminal vesicles) may have cancer in them.

Stage C1: Cancer cells have spread laterally outside the capsule.

Stage C2: Cancer cells have spread into the seminal vesicles.

Stage C3: Cancer cells have spread laterally outside the capsule and extend into the seminal vesicles.

STAGE D: Cancer cells have spread (metastasized) to lymph nodes or to organs and tissues far away from the prostate.

Stage D0: Cancer cells locally seem to be confined as indicated by a normal bone scan; however, an elevation of acid phosphatase may mean that the disease has spread to the lymph nodes (a Stage D0 may be in reality a microscopic Stage D2).

Stage D1: Cancer cells have spread to lymph nodes near the prostate. (Lymph nodes are small, bean-shaped structures that are found throughout the body. They produce and store infection-fighting cells and act as strainers.)

Stage D2: Cancer cells have spread to lymph nodes far from the prostate or to other parts of the body, such as the bone, liver, or lungs.

Stage D3: Cancer cells have spread to other parts of the body. Initial hormone therapy has failed.

The ideal staging for prostate cancer is after radical prostatectomy when the following items have been determined, however, it is my understanding that some of these tests are seldom performed by physicians. These tests are:

- PSA level
- Prostatic acid phosphatase test

- Prostatic ultrasound screening
- DNA ploidy analysis
- Lymph nodes analysis
- Bone scan
- CT scan
- MRI (optional)
- Whole mount of removed specimen

Ask Your Doctor for Your Gleason Score

Another method used by your doctor to help him or her determine the type of treatment you should get for your prostate cancer is to ascertain your Gleason scoring. The scoring of a prostate cancer tumor is accomplished either through a subjective assessment by a pathologist who assigns a Gleason grade from one to five to each of the two predominant prostate cancer cells or by a flow cytometry, which examines the genetic make-up of the individual cancer cells and assigns a grade of one to five according to their degree of malignancy.

A Gleason grade measures the state of development of cancer cells as seen through a microscope. Under the microscope, normal prostate cells are readily identifiable and are called differentiated. When cancer grows out of control, its shape loses its differentiation, mutating into five characteristic patterns. These patterns are graded from 1 to 5 on the Gleason scale, the highest number indicating less differentiation and more malignancy. A Gleason score consists of two grades of the two most prevalent patterns. For example, one of my areas of prostate cancer cells was diagnosed with a Gleason grade of 3 and the next most prevalent one with a Gleason grade of 4. Therefore, my Gleason score is 3+4 or 7, which means that it is moderately differentiated. A score of 1 to 4 indicates well-differentiated cells, 5 to 7 indicates moderate differentiation, and 8 to 10 is poorly differentiated.

Recently, when I told a colleague of mine who is in one of my support groups to ask his urologist for his Gleason score, he said that he had done so. The only comment from his doctor was, "Isn't that the name of a person [referring to Jackie Gleason, a famous television star]." The doctor was not familiar with the legitimate term! I indicated to my friend that he should get himself another doctor.

You may ask, How come I need to know so much about my prostate cancer? I personally do not think you can learn too much about a disease that may terminate your life. In addition, the more precisely your doctor is able to diagnose your condition, the better he or she will be able to recommend the most effective treatment possible.

Know the Characteristics of Your Cancer Cells

A test that is invaluable for determining if you should receive treatment for your prostate cancer or should be considered a watchful waiting patient, but which is not ordered enough by doctors, is the DNA ploidy analysis. One evening while I was attending a support group session, which consisted of nearly 100 participants, I informally asked them if anyone had ever had a DNA ploidy analysis. Much to my surprise, not a single person had heard of the study.

A flow cytometry, or more recently, MRI spectrometer blood test analysis machine, is ideal but definitely not the only criteria for determining whether a person should receive treatment or be identified as a watchful waiting candidate. A comparative analysis is made from a biopsy comparing the cancer cells to normal cells to determine the amount of DNA in the cancer cells. The ploidy analysis is done by averaging the DNA content. If the cancer cell has two sets of chromosomes, it is called diploid, which is a slowly growing cancer. If the cancer cell has more DNA than a normal cell, it is called either aneuploid or tetraploid, which are faster growing cancer cells. Other combinations that require immediate attention and treatment are any combination of aneuploid and tetraploid, which are all fast growing cells.

Research seems to indicate that 80 percent of cancer that is still confined to the prostate gland is characterized as diploid, whereas tumors that spread beyond the prostate are for the most part either aneuploid-tetraploid or aneuploid. This information is particularly useful for the urologist when a patient's disease is at Stage A or B. Stage C and D patients tend to be non-diploid.

If your tumor can be classified as either aneuploid or tetraploid, you must receive treatment immediately. If your tumor has been characterized as diploid, and depending on other factors cited in this book, you should give considerable thought to becoming a watchful waiting patient.

A recent edition of *Newsday* (May 26, 1993, pp. 20-21) reported that: "The rate of radical prostate surgery increased almost sixfold from 1984 to 1990 among American men at least 65 years old, but there is no evidence that surgery or radiation therapy is better than just waiting and monitoring patients whose cancers are in the early stages."

Dr. Craig Fleming and researchers at the Oregon Health Sciences University in Portland reviewed 144 studies in prostate cancer treatment. They found little difference in life expectancy between men who had their prostate glands removed or received radiation treatment, and those whose condition would simply be monitored by the doctors. The study found that men 65 to 70 years old who had localized prostate cancers averaged 14.1 more years of life if their cancers were merely watched, compared with 14.2 years for men who underwent radical prostatectomy (removal of the prostate gland), and 14.3 years for men who received radiation treatment.

In a survey of 304 urologists and oncologists in Canada, the United States, and Britain in 1988, each was asked what treatment they would choose if he or she was 67 years of age, diagnosed with cancer confined to the prostate gland, and had moderately differentiated prostate cancer. Of the American urologists, 79 percent said they would take surgery, while 92 percent of the radiation oncologists replied radiation. However, in Britain, where radical prostatectomy is a rarity, only 4 percent selected surgery, 44 percent opted for radiation, and the remaining percent selected watchful waiting.

Get Your Lymph Nodes Examined

If your PSA is 20.0 ng/ml or higher, you should get your lymph nodes examined to help determine the extent of your prostate cancer. Approximately 50 percent of your lymph nodes can be examined when a cyt-356 imaging agent is used with a rectal coil MRI. The other 50 percent can be examined by means of a laparoscopy.

To examine a patient's lymph nodes, Dr. Nelson Stone, a urologist at Mt. Sinai Hospital in New York City, performs a biopsy outside of the prostate gland and in the seminal vesicles prior to performing seed implantation. If there is no evidence of metastasis, he subsequently performs a lymphadenectomy, and if there is again no evidence of metastasis, he proceeds with the seed implantation.

If I could cite a weakness in my personal diagnostic study, it would be in this area: My physicians failed to recommend either of these procedures. As a result, I received external beam radiation without knowing if my disease had spread to my lymph nodes. I never knew the full extent of my prostate cancer or whether I was a stage B or C. On the other hand, my oncologist reports that if I had a laparoscopy followed by external beam radiation, I would have been at a high risk of getting lymphendema or swelling of the legs.

Know the Results of Your Other Tests

When the biopsy reveals that you have prostate cancer, your doctor should order a battery of tests to determine the extent of your cancer. He or she will usually order a bone scan to detect if the cancer has spread to your bones. He or she will also order a CT scan or MRI of your pelvis to view the tissues in your body and reveal any cancerous tumors. If these two tests do not satisfy the doctor's curiosity for one reason or another, he or she may order a skeletal survey, bone biopsy, or another bone scan, CT scan, and MRI.

For example, my doctor initially ordered a bone scan and CT scan. When the reports and film came back, the radiation

Figure 1.5
Prostate Cancer Report Card

Name: _____ Date: _____

Diagnosis/Treatment					
Diagnosis:					
Prostate Shape					
Prostate Texture					
Biopsy					
Blood Test Level (PSA)					
Prostatic Acid Phosphotase (PAP)					
Gleason Score					
Stage					
Lymph Nodes Analysis					
DNA Ploidy Analysis					
CT Scan					
Bone Scan					
Bone Biopsy					
MRI					
Skeletal Survey					
General Chemistry Serum					
Treatments:					
First					
Second					
Third					

LEGEND:

For CT Scan, Bone Scan, MRI, Lymph Nodes, Skeletal Survey:
N= Negative
P= Positive

For PSA Blood Test Level:
0 to 5,000 ng/ml

For PAP (Prostatic Acid Phosphotase):
0 - 100 ng/ml

For Gleason Rating:
MD = Moderately Differentiated

PD = Poorly Differentiated
WD = Well Differentiated

For Stages:
A_1, A_2; B_1, B_2, B_3; C_1, C_2, C_3; D_0, D_1, D_2, D_3

For DNA Ploidy Analysis:
D = Diploid
A = Aneuploid
T = Tetraploid
AT = Aneuploid/Tetraploid

Prostate Shape:
N = Normal

E = Enlarged
VE = Very Enlarged

For Prostate Texture:
H = Hard
S = Stiff
L = Lumpy
NO = Nodule
SM = Smooth
SO = Soft

General Terms:
WW = Watchful/Waiting
CHT = Combination Hormonal Treatment

RP = Radical Prostatectomy
EBR = External Beam Radiation
SI = Seed Implantation
CR = Cryosurgery
LF = Laser Fulguration
CHEMT = Chemotherapy
RT = Refractory Treatment
CT = Clinical Trial
HY = Hyperthermia

oncologist indicated that there were several spots on my bones showing either Paget's disease or carcinoma. He then ordered a bone biopsy. When he received a negative report, he ordered a survey of my entire skeleton. When that negative report was reviewed, he still was not satisfied, and thus sent me to the Memorial Sloan-Kettering Cancer Center for further study.

My doctor did not have to order all of these tests. He could have settled for utilizing only the negative results of the bone biopsy, and proceeded by recommending either an operation or radiation treatment. However, I have a people-sensitive urologist who wanted to make the best diagnosis possible in order to recommend a viable treatment for my condition.

Make Use of the Prostate Cancer Report Card

The information I have shared with you in this chapter is much too much for you to absorb in one sitting. It will take multiple readings. However, if you use my "Prostate Cancer Report Card," illustrated in Figure 1.5, you will be able to address all the items covered in this chapter with no problem. This is what you should do, after reading this chapter twice.

This chapter contains a blank copy of the Prostate Cancer Report Card. Tear it out and copy it two or three times, expanding it on your copier each time until you have a decent 8 1/2 x 11 inch version. Make several copies at this size. Next, review each item on the report card and complete the sections with which you are already familiar, guided by the legend listed at the bottom of the card. I used this card to keep track of my diagnosis and treatment. The Prostate Cancer Report Card will be of immense help to you in tracking your own prognosis and in keeping your physicians honest.

Complete My Checklist

Another technique you can use to guide you in your deliberations with your doctor is a checklist that enables you to ask your doctor pertinent questions along each step of your diagnosis and treatment. Figure 1.6 illustrates such a checklist.

Query your doctor, and when you are satisfied with his or her response to your question, check the "yes" space until you have completed the check sheet. It may be necessary for you to complete the check sheet in two sittings.

Now that you have read and absorbed this chapter, you should be familiar with certain facts about your condition, such as the size of your prostate cancer and its texture, your PSA level, your Gleason score, the stage of your cancer, and the characteristics of your prostate cancer cells. In addition, you should have information on any other tests performed to stage your condition, such as a lymph nodes analysis, CT scan, bone scan, MRI, bone biopsy, and skeletal survey. You should also know how to use the various charts in this chapter to monitor your disease. Incidentally, you should ask each of your physicians to give you a copy of each test and report he or she has on your prostate cancer condition and maintain a file on these.

Figure 1.6
Checklist for the Detection, Diagnosis, Evaluation,
and Treatment of Prostate Cancer

	YES	NO
1. As part of the regular annual physical examination, my doctor gave me a digital rectal examination by inserting a gloved finger into my rectum to determine the size and texture of my prostate gland. I asked my doctor about how it felt and its size.	_____	_____
2. Also, as part of my regular annual physical examination, my doctor gave me a blood test to determine my PSA level. I called subsequent to my examination to inquire about my PSA level. If my PSA level is over 4.0 ng/ml, I asked my doctor as to the significance of an elevated PSA level.	_____	_____
3. My doctor either felt a suspicious area on my prostate, and/or my PSA level was beyond 4.0 ng/ml. My doctor requested me to return to the office for an additional blood test. Both tests proved positive. I requested information on the next test.	_____	_____
4. I returned to my doctor's office and he or she performed a biopsy on me using a transrectal ultrasound machine. Prior to the biopsy, I asked my doctor as to how many punctures were to be made. I insist that at least three punctures were to be made. I requested my doctor explain what is seen on the screen.	_____	_____
5. When the information on the biopsy was received by my doctor, he or she requested me to appear in his or her office for consultation. I asked him or her to explain the findings of the biopsy and explain the next step.	_____	_____

Figure 1.6 (Continued)
Checklist for the Detection, Diagnosis, Evaluation,
and Treatment of Prostate Cancer

		YES	NO
6.	My doctor stated that the biopsy was either negative or positive. If positve, I asked my doctor to inform me of my Gleason grade and stage. I also requested my doctor to report the DNA characteristic of my prostate. We discussed the next step. My doctor ordered a lymph node analysis, CT scan, bone scan, MRI, and X-ray to further illuminate the stage of my prostate cancer. I requested that my doctor debulk and downstage my cancer with combination hormonal therapy if I had an enlarged prostate gland. I also asked my doctor to evaluate my lymph nodes for cancer, and he or she agreed.	_____	_____
7.	I returned to my doctor's office and he or she explained the results of the various tests. If my doctor ordered new tests, I requested him or her to explain the reasons and results.	_____	_____
8.	The results of any new tests were discussed. I requested my doctor to explain all the traditional treatments, side effects, and what I could expect, and to do so for all nontraditional treatments. I asked my doctor to give me his or her recommendation and state the reasons.	_____	_____
9.	I explained my doctor's choice of treatment and the reasons to my family. I considered my doctor's choice of treatments and reasons thereof as well as all the traditional and non traditional treatments. I decided on a treatment and discussed it with my family.	_____	_____
10.	I returned to my doctor's office and indicated that I agreed or disagreed with his or her choice of options and I indicated why. I asked my doctor if he or she would go along with my choice of option(s) and he or she consented or dissented.	_____	_____
11.	I asked all my doctors for copies of my records and made them available to the doctor(s) treating me.	_____	_____
12.	My doctor and I reached a mutual agreement on a contingency plan in the event of a recurrence of my disease.	_____	_____

CHAPTER TWO

Understanding Your Choices of Treatment for Prostate Cancer

There are more than six treatments for prostate cancer. A few have stood the test of time and have been verified as effective to varying degrees through five- and ten-year statistical survival studies. Other treatments have yet to be proven effective over an extended period of time. Some have proven ineffective in the past in terms of long-term survival. However, today these same treatments are beginning to show promising results because of new procedures and modern medical technology, such as the transrectal ultrasound machine, interactive computers, and other equipment. Furthermore, some physicians are experiencing more success with some forms of treatment because they are giving their patients combination hormonal therapy as a preliminary therapy to shrink the prostate gland in order to make it more manageable for treatment. Some of these same doctors are following up with external beam radiation if there is a suspicion of any residual disease. And some physicians are retreating their patients with the same treatment if the initial treatment failed to rid the patient of all of the disease.

If you are considering treatments for prostate cancer, you have two choices, the traditional pathway or the nontraditional pathway. With the traditional pathway, you can decide to select from among traditional or standard treatments, such as radical

prostatectomy, external beam radiation, or bilateral orchiectomy (removal of the testes). With nontraditional, you can decide to select from among several nontraditional or
nonstandard treatments, such as cryosurgery, seed implantation, hyperthermia, laser fulguration, combination hormonal
therapy, and chemotherapy.

There are several advantages of the traditional treatments
over the nontraditional treatments:

- Both radical prostatectomy and external beam radiation
  have ten-year statistical survival studies.

- Traditional treatments are less risky in terms of survival.

- More trained physicians practice the traditional treatments.

- More hospitals provide these treatments.

- Insurance companies will reimburse patients for medical costs.

There are also some advantages of the nontraditional treatments over the traditional treatments:

- They are not as invasive.

- It usually takes less time to complete the treatment.

- The treatments are less costly, however, insurance companies may not reimburse patients for undergoing nontraditional treatments for prostate cancer.

- The recuperative time is less.

- The side effects are usually minimal.

- Modern medical technology has increased the efficacy
  of many of these treatments.

- No mortality rate has been reported.

- Blood loss is kept at a minimum.

While the nontraditional pathway for treating prostate cancer may seem to be more inviting because of minimal side
effects and the short treatment and recovery span, they may

pose more of a risk because they have not been proven in either five or ten-year statistical survival studies.

TRADITIONAL PATHWAY FOR TREATING PROSTATE CANCER

As I indicated, the term traditional refers to generally accepted standard treatments that have stood the test over a period of five- and ten-year statistical survival studies. Below I will explain each of the treatments.

Radical Prostatectomy

Radical prostatectomy—surgical removal of the cancerous prostate gland—is considered to be the gold standard for prostate cancer in the United States, that is, this is not necessarily so in other countries. Recently, in some instances, radical prostatectomy has been preceded by combination hormonal therapy to make the gland more manageable for treatment and sometimes succeeded by external beam radiation if there is some suspicion of any marginal cancer based on the surgery.

There are primarily two surgical approaches to prostate cancer: the retropubic approach and the radical perineal prostatectomy. In the retropubic approach, a vertical incision is made along the midline of the abdomen, from the navel to the pubic bone, and lymph nodes are removed for pathological study. A determination is then made whether to proceed or not to proceed with the operation. This should be discussed and agreed to by the patient and his doctor before the operation.

Stephen N. Rous, M.D., author of *The Prostate Book* (Consumer Reports Books, Yonkers, NY: 1992, pp. 171-172), cogently describes this surgical approach:

A long up-and-down incision is made in the midline of the abdomen from the navel to the pubic bone. After the lymph nodes have been removed for study by the pathologist and a determination has been made to proceed with the removal of the prostate gland, the space underneath the pubic bone is cleaned and dissected and the removal of the entire prostate gland is generally begun at the end that is farthest from the bladder, next to the external urethral sphincter. The prostatic urethra is divided at the point; then it and the prostate gland through which it goes are pulled upwards toward the bladder while the dissection continues behind the prostate gland, separating it from the layer of tissue that is connected to the rectum on its other side. As the dissection continues between the prostate and the rectum, the seminal vesicles, which are behind the base of the bladder, come into view and will be removed along with the prostate gland. This dissection of the seminal vesicles from the back wall of the bladder is generally done after the bladder neck has been cut across. Once the seminal vesicles are free, the entire prostate gland and the seminal vesicles are removed. The bladder neck is then stitched closed to a small enough diameter so that it is about the same size as the stump of the urethra from which the prostate was detached. The bladder neck is then pulled down into the pelvis and snuggled up against the urethral stump and stitched to it. This stitching is done around a Foley catheter which has been inserted through the penis all the way into the bladder.

When considering this surgical approach, bear in mind the following:

- The lymph nodes and prostate gland can be removed at the same time.

- Recuperation as a result of the abdominal incision creates more of a hardship for patients.

- Infection is possible.

- There is a 60 percent chance that you will become incontinent (inability to control your urine after the operation); and a 3 percent risk of permanent incontinence.

- You also stand a 5 percent chance of cardiopulmonary troubles and rectal or bowel injury.

- There is a possibility of a great amount of blood loss.

- According to Medicare data, 1 percent of men below the age of 65 to 74 who receive this treatment for prostate cancer have died of this procedure and 2 percent of the men aged 75 and older have died of this procedure.

- This same document reports 60 to 90 percent of the men were impotent as a result of this procedure.

- You will require a six- or seven-day hospital confinement.

- Your recovery period is six months to two years.

- This treatment is not applicable if the disease has progressed beyond the prostate gland.

- There is a high failure rate due to understaging the prostate cancer patient.

- This is a very expensive treatment.

- This treatment requires prior laparoscopy or lymphadenectomy to examine the patient's lymph nodes.

- Either general or local anesthesia is required.

The second alternative surgical procedure for prostate cancer is through the perineum, which is the area between the scrotum and the anus. Dr. Rous continues by describing the radical perineal prostatectomy on p. 176 of his book:

The surgical incision that is used for a radical perineal prostatectomy is usually in the shape of an inverted "U" going right over the anus, with the center of the U about three centimeters above the margin of the anus. In extending the incision deeply into the tissues of the perineum, it is important to release the attachments of the rectum to the urethra so that the rectum will fall away towards the back of the patient while the urethra and ultimately the prostate gland are more anterior, thereby minimizing the chance of damaging the rectum. The prostate gland is freed from its surrounding structures by gentle dissection, and the urethra at the end of the prostate farthest from the bladder is isolated and divided. The bladder neck is freed from the prostate, and, once the prostate gland has been removed and the bladder neck has been closed sufficiently so that the size of its opening approximates the size of the urethral opening, the urethra and the bladder neck are stitched together. A catheter is left in place postoperatively for about two weeks.

In addition to the various complications cited for the retropubic approach, the following are some complications that may occur with the radical perineal approach:

- This procedure is more suitable for prostate cancer patients with heart problems and it is faster than the retropubic approach.

- Urethral structure damage occurs in 7 percent of the patients.

- There is a likelihood for two operations: one for removal of the lymph nodes and one for removal of the prostate gland and seminal vesicles.

External Beam Radiation Therapy

In external beam radiation therapy, the prostate is subject to a brief period of bombardment by a focused beam of X-rays from a machine. The intent of the X-rays is to shrink the cancerous tumor or to destroy the ability of the cancer cells to grow and divide. The equipment can either be the low energy protons cobalt-60 unit, or the linear accelerator (which was used on me). My radiation oncologist, George Varsos, M.D., maintains that radiation treatment to the pelvis using anything but a high energy linear accelerator will cause a higher incidence of complications and that no prostate cancer patients should undergo definitive treatment with low energy protons or a cobalt-60 unit.

The patient usually goes to the hospital for seven to eight weeks and receives no more than 200 rads per session for a total of 6,000 to 7,200 rads to minimize damage to normal tissue. (A rad or centigram is a unit of measurement of the amount of radiation received.) I received 6,800 rads over 33 treatments. Each treatment lasts from 3 to 5 minutes and is painless. However, treatment is not started until the area has been identified through a "simulation" exercise in which the treatment area is marked with indelible ink for whites and white out for blacks. These marks are to ensure that the identical area is treated every time. Studies show that the success rate over a ten-year period for radical prostatectomy and external beam radiation therapy appears to be the same, with a slight edge for radical prostatectomy.

If you decide on external beam radiation therapy as your treatment of choice, you should consider the following:

- Use combination hormonal therapy to debulk and downstage your prostate to make it more manageable for treatment.
- It frequently shows a disturbing presence of persistent prostate cancer six months or more after treatment.
- Urinary obstructions may exist for 10 to 15 percent of patients.
- Near the end of the treatment, the patient may begin to feel tired.
- Your treatment requires six to eight weeks.
- Healthy cells are also damaged in the process of killing prostate cancer cells.
- This is a very expensive treatment.
- The success rate seems to be increasing when the three-dimensional radiation imaging is used.
- It causes chronic diarrhea in 5 percent of patients.

- Sometimes this treatment is used as a salvage treatment when marginal disease is suspected.

- There is a 50 percent probability of impotence after treatment.

- May cause severe bladder size reduction.

- May cause rectal sphincter damage and accompanying rectal incontinence.

- May cause prostate scar tissue, constricting the urethra and thus restricting urinary flow.

Do not be afraid of the litany of aftereffects of external beam radiation therapy. Most of these did not affect me or most of the colleagues in my support groups. The five- and ten-year survival statistical studies for radiation therapy is about 90 percent for Stage A, 80 percent for Stage B, and 35 to 40 percent for Stage C. These statistics are very similar to radical prostatectomy. However, a major difference between the two therapies is that usually after surgery, there is little evidence of cancer, whereas with external beam radiation, some studies report that more than 50 percent of patients continue to have cancer in the prostate gland. I personally believe these figures are likely to change when radiation therapy is succeeded after three to six months of combination hormonal therapy.

Bilateral Orchiectomy

The vast majority of the prostate cancer cells are dependent on testosterone to grow. One method used by physicians to decrease testosterone in the body is the removal of the primary source of testosterone, the testes. It should be understood that the reduction of circulating testosterone to nearly zero level slows down the rate of growth of prostate cancer cells. Although this technique is not a cure for prostate cancer, it is a traditional treatment that has been used by physicians for years to palliate (to lessen the effects of testosterone in the body) prostate cancer.

If bilateral orchiectomy is your choice of treatment, you should consider the following:

- This therapy is identified as the gold standard for decreasing the production of testosterone in the body.

- It is inexpensive.

- Usually, flutamide or a substitute is administered with this treatment.

- Several studies report that its efficacy in decreasing testosterone in the body is not as successful as combination hormonal therapy.

- Ninety percent of circulating testosterone is secreted by the testes and 5 to 10 percent of circulating testosterone is secreted by the adrenal glands. However, when the testes are removed, Fernand Labrie, M.D. of Laval University in Quebec, Canada, maintains that the adrenal glands may contribute up to 40 percent of the testosterone within the prostate cancer cells.

- Impotence occurs in 95 percent of patients.

- This procedure is irreversible and may permanently affect the functioning of the body's immune system.

- This procedure is not a cure for prostate cancer.

- This therapy is appropriate for you if your disease has spread to your lymph nodes, bones, or elsewhere in your body.

- This procedure has two distinct advantages over combination hormonal therapy in that you do not have to continually administer the treatment and do not have to take any medication.

- Some practitioners claim that testosterone levels drop by 90 to 95 percent, immediately decreasing the supply to the prostate cancer cells.

- You do not have to take injections for the duration of your treatment.

- This procedure can be performed under either local or general anesthetic and has few risks in general.
- Zoladex or luprolide can be substituted for surgical castration.
- Flutamide should always be taken with bilateral orchiectomy.

At times, physicians have prescribed high doses of estrogen as a substitute for surgical castration to block the formation of androgens by the testes. However, because of its severe side effects, such as 15 percent of the patients dying within one year of treatment, this technique has been abandoned by some contemporary physicians.

NONTRADITIONAL PATHWAY
FOR TREATING PROSTATE CANCER

PAACT maintains that combination hormonal therapy is the gold standard for the treatment of all stages of prostate cancer regardless of the stage. Although I believe this to be true because combination hormonal therapy was used to debulk my prostate and decrease my PSA level from 41.0 ng/ml to 0 ng/ml over a period of several months, I could find no other sources that make this claim. In addition, my radiation oncologist maintains that combination hormonal therapy has not been proven in any study to add to the disease-free or overall survival in those patients with minimal, nonbulky prostate cancer.

Throughout this book, I will recommend combination hormonal therapy as a preliminary treatment for most stages of prostate cancer based on my review of the research of Dr. Labrie and others on combination hormonal therapy, PAACT's recommendation, and my personal experience with this type of therapy. Should you request your physician to prescribe combination hormonal therapy as a preliminary treatment for your prostate cancer? I say, absolutely, yes! I admit my bias. However, the choice is left to you and not your physician. Not all patients are "cured" with traditional therapy and some traditional treatments may have more side effects than are desired.

For these reasons, nontraditional or investigative treatments, or clinical trials based on the most up-to-date information are designed to find better ways to treat cancer patients.

Cryosurgery

Cryosurgery, or freezing of the prostate gland, is not new and is presently used as an experimental treatment. In fact, it was first used about thirty years ago. However, because of severe side effects, it was abandoned. With the advent of transrectal ultrasound technology, however, it has reemerged as a viable technique and an alternative to radical prostatectomy. In a two-hour procedure under general anesthesia, cryosurgery is performed by freezing the prostate gland using liquid nitrogen which is circulated in small tubes called cryoprobes. Ultrasound is used to monitor the cryosurgical procedure.

If cryosurgery is your treatment of choice, consider the following:

- Use combination hormonal therapy for six months to debulk and downstage your disease to increase the likelihood of maximum success.

- In a national study, 6.1 percent of patients' rectums also were frozen.

- It is less costly than radical prostatectomy and external beam radiation.

- It can be performed as an outpatient procedure and usually takes two to three hours to complete.

- Efficiency is increased due to the transrectal ultrasound machine.

- It is currently applicable for early-staged patients; some success is being realized with late-staged patients.

- There is no or limited blood loss.

- There is less incontinence and/or impotence than with traditional treatments.

- There is no need for surgical incision.

- It is ideally suited for patients with other medical problems.
- There was some deadening of prostate urethral tissue in 4 to 5 percent of the patients.
- There are no five- and ten-year survival statistics on the procedure of cryosurgery.
- It may be repeated if the initial treatment is unsuccessful or if marginal disease is detected after the procedure is completed.

Brachytherapy

The term brachytherapy means short-distant therapy. Some practitioners use the term whenever they are talking about internal radiation therapy. One form of brachytherapy is Iodine-125 seed implantation:

A booklet distributed by Amsterdam Healthcare, entitled "Another Therapeutic Approach to Prostate Cancer: Radioactive Seed Implantation," vividly describes I-125 seed implantation.

Under this method of therapy, tiny pellets containing radioactive medication, such as Iodine-125 seeds, are permanently implanted directly in the middle of the cancer where they give off low level radiation continuously for approximately one year. Using TURP guidance, these seeds are positioned so that radiation is distributed throughout the prostate gland. Since only a small area is radiated by each seed, relatively little radiation reaches the adjacent normal organs. The implant procedure does not require a surgical incision. Instead, the seeds—smaller than grains of rice—are contained in thin needles which are passed into the prostate gland through the skin between the scrotum and rectum. As the seeds penetrate through the prostate, they are seen on the screen of the ultrasound machine and can be accurately guided to their final position. While the needles are being inserted the ultrasound probe is in the rectum. When each needle is in its correct position in the prostate, the needle is slowly withdrawn and the individual seeds are injected into the prostate gland. The ultrasound probe and the needles are removed when the procedure has been completed. The numbers of needles and seeds required varies from patient to patient depending on the size of the prostate gland.

If you choose I-125 seed implantation as your treatment, you should consider the following:

- Use combination hormonal therapy for six months to debulk and downstage your disease to increase the likelihood of maximum success.

- The best results occur when an ultrasound machine is used to depict a three-dimensional image of the prostate.

- There is no long-term incontinence.

- Seed implantation has an improved side effects profile over other treatments.

- It is less costly than radical prostatectomy or external beam radiation.

- John Blasko, M.D., a radiation oncologist at the Northwest Tumor Institute in Seattle, Washington, who started I-125 seed implantation in 1985, reports that eight years of experience with this treatment show that more than 90 percent of the patients are free of prostate cancer and have an immeasurable PSA for 2 to 4 years. However, my radiation oncologist claims that the technique has not proven to be as effective in irradiating the tumor, though I have recommended this treatment for an old time friend who is 69 years of age and did not want surgery or external beam radiation.

- A procedure that combines ultrasound and fluoroscopy should be used to visually show internal radiation therapy to achieve a satisfactory prostate distribution of I-125 seeds.

- An interactive computer and patient follow up by CT scan should be used to assure accurate seed placement and distribution, which is critical to treatment success.
- This procedure cannot be repeated.
- This procedure is sometimes accompanied by external beam radiation.
- It does not necessitate hospital confinement and usually takes two to three hours to complete the procedure.
- It does not require general anesthesia.
- Usually this treatment is applicable with early-staged patients.
- Patients with early Stage A and B and small prostate tumors are the best candidates.
- The most recent clinical data, based on 451 patients followed for up to six years, shows a higher percentage of implant patients remaining disease-free than with either radical prostatectomy or external beam therapy.
- Because they are placed at the site of the cancer, the seeds can deliver two or three times more concentrated radiation to the prostate gland than external radiation therapy, which must use a lower dose because it also affects healthy tissue.

Seed implants are not only done with Iodine-125, but are also done with palladium-103 seeds. In fact, palladium has advantages over Iodine-125 because it has a higher radiation dose with a much shorter life span; however, it is about five times more expensive, and most of the research available has been done on Iodine-125.

Laser Fulguration

Laser fulguration is also a form of brachytherapy. It is a two-stage process. In stage one, a transrectal ultrasound of the prostate is made whereby soundwave echoes are used to create an image of the prostate to visually inspect any abnormal conditions. After about three to five weeks of the extensive TURP, stage two is completed. Stage two involves the use of laser irradiation guided under transrectal ultrasound observation and guidance. This procedure is based on the concept that the bulk of the cancerous prostate tumor is removed by electroresection, and then remnants of the cancerous tumor near the capsule or cover of the prostate could be destroyed by laser coagulation.

If laser fulguration is your treatment of choice, consider the following:

- There are no five- and ten-year survival statistics.

- There are probably other side effects, but I have not been able to determine these.

Hyperthermia

The rationale behind hyperthermia, or treatment of the prostate with heat, is that when heat is applied to the prostate gland, it will shrink and the cancer cells will be destroyed. The heat is delivered at a temperature of 42 to 55 degrees centigrade, either up against the prostate or in the prostate. The heat is generated by a machine. One such machine is the Prostatron. The heat is applied one time over a period of 30 to 60 minutes depending on the size of the prostate gland. The procedure is conducted under local anesthetic and no hospitalization is required. Hyperthermia has been used in Europe for some time and is being used by a few cancer centers in the United States.

Usually six treatments of one hour each are given over a period of weeks during which time you can lead a normal life. You will usually suffer no more than a slight discomfort from the catheterization for each treatment. The temperature is very accurately controlled by a thermocouple situated in a catheter in the prostatic urethra which is connected to a personal computer that directs and monitors the entire process. Some prostate cancer patients are unsuitable for hyperthermia treatment such as those who have bladder or prostatic stones; those whose prostate gland is too small or too big; those who have any abnormalities of the urethra; and those who have had rectal surgery except for piles.

Since this treatment has limited use in the United States, I do not have access to all of the data regarding its advantages and disadvantages. However, if hyperthermia is your treatment of choice, consider the following:

- It is performed only in a few centers in this country.
- There are no five- and ten-year survival statistic studies.
- Few physicians are trained in this process.
- It requires very expensive equipment.
- There is less research on this treatment than with some of the other nontraditional treatments.
- It is not as popular among physicians as some of the other treatments.

Proton Beam Radiation

With this treatment, proton beam radiation is converged on a very selective apex that is able to precisely focus on a prostate cancer tumor and deliver the therapeutic rays without damaging the normal tissue to treat the malignant tumor. Due to the high degree of selectivity, higher doses of radiation can be administered with less harsh effects to adjacent tissue. There are also fewer and milder side effects.

If you choose this treatment, you should consider the following:

- There are no five- and ten-year statistical survival studies.
- The equipment is expensive and there is only one hospital I know of that has it (Loma Linda University Medical Center in Loma Linda, California).
- This treatment reduces nerve compression and is useful for treating pain.

- Only a few doctors in this country are trained in this treatment.
- This treatment is usually only viable for Stage A and B patients.
- Consider using three to six months of hormonal therapy prior to this treatment to debulk an enlarged cancerous prostate gland.

Combination Hormonal Therapy

Recently, two major discoveries have been made regarding a substitute for surgical castration and a replacement for estrogen by the Medical Research Council Group in Molecular Endocrinology at the Laval Medical Center in Quebec, Canada. The first discovery involves the administration of a hormone agonist to block testosterone produced by the testes technically referred to as Luteinizing Hormone Releasing Hormone (LHRH agonist). This hormone agonist is administered every twenty-nine days through an injection in the buttock, arm, or in a muscle in the abdomen. Some LHRH agonists are luprolide, zoladex, or buserelin (the latter has not been approved by the Food and Drug Administration or FDA). The second important discovery involves the administration of a pure antiandrogen to be used in combination with the LHRH agonist to block androgens at the receptor sites in the prostate cancer cells. This antiandrogen is taken three times per day every eight hours for the entire treatment period and can be prescribed under the title of flutamide, casodex, nilutamide or cyproterone acetate (the latter three have not been approved by the FDA).

If combination therapy is your choice of treatment, you should consider the following:

- Use this therapy as a preliminary treatment for most stages of your prostate cancer. Although combination hormonal therapy has been shown to increase the efficacy of external beam radiation treatment in bulkier disease, my radiation oncologist indicates that there appears to be little if any advantage to the use of combination hormonal therapy with small prostate cancer tumors.

- This treatment will require an injection in your buttock (luprolide) or an injection in the subcutaneous tissue of your abdomen of a hormone (zoladex) every month and two pills of flutamide at 125 mg each every eight hours daily.

- The medication is very expensive, costing a combined yearly total of about $8,000; however, medicare will cover luprolide and zoladex if you are eligible as will most insurance companies.

- This therapy is used quite often to debulk and downstage the prostate in order to make the gland more manageable for treatment.

- This treatment is at times mandatory for patients with advanced stage prostate cancer.

- This therapy usually fails when the prostate cancer cells are no longer dependent on androgens.

- Hot flashes associated with flutamide may be controlled with an injection of Depo-Provera, tablets of Megace, clonidine, or dose reduction.

- Diarrhea may be controlled with Imodium-AD or by substituting flutamide with cyproterone acetate, which is not available in the United States.

- Chronic use of combination hormonal therapy may result in decreased chest and shoulder muscle mass.

- Indigestion occurs in some patients who are taking flutamide. However, this can usually be eliminated if it is taken with food and/or the dosage is reduced.

- When this treatment is continued and the PSA level continues to rise, there probably is a recurrence of prostate cancer.

- This therapy usually drastically reduces PSA levels to values of less than 1.0 ng/ml.

- Associated pain may be controlled by radioisotopes such as Metastron (or samarium), which is not available in the United States.

- Impotence occurs in nearly all cases; sexual function may return when the therapy is discontinued.

- Liver problems including jaundice rarely occur.

Chemotherapy

When combination hormonal therapy, consisting of luprolide and flutamide, fails to arrest your prostate cancer, your physician should consider using other hormones and/or drugs to arrest your disease, such as those cited in this book. When all else fails and a reevaluation proves predominant presence of androgen-independent cells, you and your physician's next option is chemotherapy. Chemotherapy involves the administration of highly potent chemicals to the patient with prostate cancer to diminish or halt cancer growth in the body. When such chemicals are ingested, they harm both healthy and unhealthy cells. However, the greater harm is to those cells that grow the fastest, which are usually cancerous cells and those responsible for growing hair. Although there are numerous drugs being used to treat prostate cancer, none have been very effective. One problem seems to be the ability of the drug to reach the prostate through the bloodstream.

A promising new drug is suramin, which is technologically not a true chemotherapeutic agent. In order for cells to divide into cancerous and healthy cells, they need growth factors. Prostate cancer cells respond excessively to these growth factors and suramin somehow interferes with them and therefore halts the cancerous cells from growing.

If you consider this drug as your choice of treatment, you should give serious attention to the following:

- There are no available five- or ten-year survival statistic studies.

- It can cause infections, rashes, and damage to the nervous system.
- It is generally unavailable except for a few clinical trials.
- It may destroy the adrenal glands.
- Chemotherapy can cause blood problems, such as abnormalities in clotting mechanisms.
- There are a multitude of side effects, such as nausea, fatigue, bodily pain, and hair loss.

Other Drugs

Below are other drugs that deserve consideration.

CYTADREN: This drug prevents adrenal androgen secretion. When administered with low-dose hydrocortisone replacement, it is effective with a survival probability of 50 percent at 21 months for those patients who are responsive to the drug.

NIZORAL: This drug was developed for fungal infections. It has been known to inhibit testicular and adrenal androgen production when used in high dosage. It has also been effective as a therapeutic value in the treatment of some advanced stage patients with prostate cancer.

DIPHOSPHONATES: This drug has been found to be effective to some degree in dealing with bone pain in prostate cancer patients.

CASODEX and CYPROTERONE ACETATE: These drugs are antiandrogens and may be effective for those prostate cancer patients who are unable to tolerate, or are nonresponsive to flutamide. Casodex is reported to block testosterone action without causing impotence.

Radiopharmaceuticals for Prostate Cancer

About 50 percent of prostate cancer spreads to the bones. Decreasing pain from these lesions is important to a patient's quality of life. Although radiation also does have some propensity to reduce bone pain in patients with prostate cancer, it also has some effects on a patient's bone marrow and can limit his ability to function properly.

Recently there has been increased use of radiopharmaceuticals for bone pain relief in patients with advanced prostate cancer (those with Stage D2 disease in the bone). One of the most promising of the radiopharmaceuticals for pain is the strontium-89 chloride injection known as Metastron. Strontium-89 is a metal that can form a salt that is able to be dissolved in the blood plasma. The strontium emits a low energy electron that irradiates tissue. This electron has a very short travel range. Therefore, only areas that are microscopically close to the dissolved strontium will take the radiation. The strontium is very similar to calcium, and is absorbed in the bones by areas that are being broken down by the tumor.

One clinical trial demonstrated the efficacy of strontium-89 when patients with advanced prostate cancer, who were treated in one site of the bone with external beam radiation followed up with strontium-89 treatment, showed a delayed onset of further metastases. Strontium-89 has also been found to be effective at earlier stages of the disease, as well as in delaying the progression of pain. Although it is not associated with any significant survival benefits, it is 80 percent effective in decreasing pain.

If one or more of these chemotherapies is your treatment of choice, you should consider the following:

- There are no five- or ten-year survival statistic studies.
- There may be mild blood problems as a result.
- There may be some transient pain, though it is mild and controllable.

No Treatment (Watchful Waiting)

There is considerable evidence that if your prostate cancer has been diagnosed as a Stage A or B and you meet certain other criteria such as age, that it may be more beneficial for you to become a watchful waiting patient. Studies in Sweden and Britain show that there is very little difference in the mortality rate for men who have undergone radical prostatectomy and those who accepted watchful waiting as their approach to the disease. In fact, some physicians maintain that men over the age of 70 stand a good chance of dying of something other than prostate cancer. However, if you and your doctor opt for watchful waiting, I strongly recommend that your disease be monitored very carefully.

An effective way to do this is to develop a contingency plan for prostate cancer that contains trigger points, as indicated in Figure 2.1.

Dynamic Monitoring

Another method you may wish to consider is referred to as dynamic monitoring whereby your PSA level is taken on a monthly basis. After six months, a biopsy is performed in which a minimum of six punctures are conducted to look for any progression of the disease.

Figure 2.1
Contingency Plan for Prostate Cancer

Treatment Strategy	Date	Trigger Point	New Treatment Strategy
1. Watchful waiting patient	June 1994	PSA level remains below 6	Do nothing but monitor carefully
2. Take new blood test	Continue this process every 3 months	PSA level between 7 and 10	Take a new biopsy; look for increased tumor size and Gleason score
3. Reconsider traditional and nontraditional treatments	When deemed necessary	Pathology report indicates tumor size has increased by 20% and Gleason score has increased to 5 or more	Take combination hormonal therapy for 6 months followed by cryosurgery

Which Pathway Should You Choose?

The previous contents of this chapter described both the traditional and nontraditional pathways for treating prostate cancer. Which type of treatment you select will be based on the following factors:

- Your personality, that is, if you are risk-oriented and favor an investigative approach, or if you are conservative and favor a conservative approach, one that has five- and ten-year survival statistic studies.

- You may leave the decision entirely in your doctor's hands.

- The bias of your preference based on what you have learned.

- It may depend on the type of doctor you go to. For example, if you seek a urologist, he or she may recommend radical prostatectomy. If you go to a radiation oncologist, he or she may recommend external beam radiation.

- You may base your decision on your own comprehensive research study that led to either a traditional or a nontraditional approach.

- Your sexual activities may be the basis for making a decision. A member of one of my support groups who is in his early seventies decided to do nothing but rely on nutrition to accommodate his condition so he could continue an active sexual life.

- Your decision may be based on interviews with numerous patients who undergo both traditional and nontraditional methods of treatment for their prostate cancer. Another member of my prostate cancer support group made contact with ten patients who had radical prostatectomies and external beam radiation. Several of those who underwent a radical prostatectomy were still suffering side effects two years after the operation. Those who had the radiation were experiencing very little side effects. My colleague settled for radiation.

- You may decide to discuss the side effects with members of your family and to reach a consensus with them about the best decision.

- Your quality of life may be a factor when considering a treatment for prostate cancer. For example, a person who is seriously interested in continuing an active sexual life might resist either radical prostatectomy or external beam radiation and opt instead for seed implantation.

A member of my support group was scheduled to undergo a radical prostatectomy until he conducted a comprehensive study. He had numerous conversations with doctors and prostate cancer patients and finally decided on cryosurgery to treat his prostate cancer. Take your time when making a decision about your choice of treatment.

TREATMENT BY CELL TYPE/STAGE

Previously, I presented the various treatments for prostate cancer. In this section, I will associate these treatments with the various stages. These are indicated for patients to discuss with their physicians and arrive at a mutual choice for treatment.

Stage A: Pathological Stage

Stage A disease is confined to the prostate gland. The PSA level may be slightly elevated, the Gleason score is 2 to 4; and the tumor is well-differentiated.

Stage A1: Disease has one, two, or three sites of well-differentiated tumors or less than 5 percent of the volume of tissue removed.

Stage A2: Disease has more than three well-differentiated tumors or any quantity of higher grade tumor or more than 5 percent of the volume of tissue removed.

If you have been diagnosed as Stage A, you should consider one or more of the following to treat your disease:

1. Watchful waiting.
2. Begin with six months of combination hormonal therapy. However, one of my reviewers indicated that he would not recommend this treatment to his Stage A patients. Consult your doctor.
3. Get a radical prostatectomy followed by external beam radiation if there is clinical evidence that the disease has spread beyond the margin of surgery.
4. Receive external beam radiation.
5. Consider cryosurgery, hyperthermia, laser fulguration, seed implantation, or proton beam irradiation.
6. Repeat cryosurgery using the transrectal ultrasound machine when external beam radiation failed to eliminate all of the cancer.
7. Repeat cryosurgery if the first attempt at cryosurgery fails.

Stage B: Clinical Stage

Stage B disease clinically is confined to the prostate by rectal digital examination and is confirmed by a transrectal examination and biopsy.

Stage B1: Disease occupies less than one lobe and is less than 1.5 cm in diameter.

Stage B2: Disease occupies one entire lobe or both lobes or bilateral nodules and is more than 1.5 cm in diameter.

Stage B3: Disease occupies bilateral nodules.

If you have been diagnosed as Stage B, you should consider one or more of the following to treat your disease:

1. Begin with six months of combination hormonal therapy.
2. Get a radical prostatectomy followed by external beam radiation if there is clinical evidence of marginal disease.
3. Receive external beam radiation.
4. Consider cryosurgery, hyperthermia, laser fulguration, seed implantation, or proton beam irradiation.

5. Receive cryosurgery using transrectal ultrasound machine if external beam radiation failed to eliminate all of the cancer.

6. Repeat cryosurgery if the first attempt at cryosurgery fails.

Stage C: Clinical Stage

Stage C disease clinically is usually confined locally, but the lesion of the prostate extends laterally outside the prostate or into the seminal vesicles. Treatment for these stages of the disease should be to control the growth of the cancerous tumor, prevent movement of malignant cells to other parts of the body, and maximize the period in which you are free from any unpleasant consequences of the disease.

Stage C1: Disease has lateral extension.

Stage C2: Disease has seminal vesicle extension.

Stage C3: Disease has both extensions.

If you have been diagnosed as Stage C, you should consider one or more of the following to treat your prostate cancer condition:

1. Begin with combination hormonal therapy for a period of six months to debulk the volume of the tumor and downstage the disease to make it more manageable, followed by external beam radiation.

2. Consider radical prostatectomy if there is no lymph node involvement.

3. Consider cryosurgery, seed implantation, or laser fulguration using the transrectal ultrasound machine.

Stage D: Imaging, Biochemical Stage

Treatments for these stages are directed toward prolonging life by preventing further spread of the disease and providing relief from symptoms of the disease.

Stage D0: Disease is clinically locally confined with normal bone scan, but may have metastasized.

Stage D1: Disease is locally confined within invaded pelvic lymph nodes.

Stage D2: Disease has spread to any of the following: the bones; soft tissue; lymph nodes; lungs; or liver.

Stage D3: Combination hormonal therapy is no longer effective.

If you have been diagnosed as Stage D, you and your physician should consider either one or a combination of the following:

1. Begin with a minimum of six months of combination hormonal therapy (luprolide and flutamide), however, one of my reviewers maintains that he would not prescribe this treatment.
2. Get a radical prostatectomy (as recommended by Dr. Rous) followed by external beam radiation only if you have been diagnosed with stage D1. However, one of my reviewers indicated that he would not recommend this treatment to his patients.
3. Continue combination hormonal therapy if luprolide and flutamide are no longer effective, using cytadren 250 mg every 6 hours, and low-dose hydrocortisone acetate (10 mg morning, 5 mg afternoon, and 5 mg in the evening).
4. Use combination emcyt/velban (six weeks of both drugs then four times a week) if combination hormonal therapy is no longer effective and you do not have bone marrow impairment.
5. Try radiopharmaceuticals, such as strontium-89 in combination with cis-platinum.

I will not tell you how you should make treatment decisions. I will advise you from my personal experience and the extensive research I have completed to consider the following:

1. Thoroughly study both traditional and nontraditional pathways for treating prostate cancer.
2. Know the side effects of all treatments.

3. Talk to patients who have undergone various traditional and nontraditional treatments.

4. Talk to a physician (this usually means an oncologist) who is well-versed in the treatment of advanced prostate cancer.

5. Be aware of your own condition. This should be used as a strong platform for helping you to make a treatment decision.

6. Consider developing a contingency treatment plan should your first choice of treatment fail.

If you are like the thousands of men who were informed by their physicians that they have prostate cancer, you will no doubt find the literature on prostate cancer, as well as various doctors' opinions of this disease very confusing. In fact, the more you read about prostate cancer, the more confused you will become. My only suggestions to you are to learn as much as you can about your particular stage, seek out others who have a similar stage and learn from them, and seek the opinions of three (not two) other doctors. Do not confine your research to studies in the United States either, but consider studies in Canada, Britain, and other countries.

CHAPTER THREE

Some Questionable Practices I Discovered in the Diagnosis and Treatment Of Prostate Cancer

I felt a strong need to write this chapter because of what I learned through my research, readings, and interactions with numerous doctors, and with hundreds of patients who have prostate cancer. True, my doctorate is in philosophy, not medicine; however, physicians who were kind and assisted me with this book agreed with me to some degree, or these practices would not be discussed here. Some of these practices no doubt have either caused problems for prostate cancer patients, reduced their longevity, or actually led to their deaths. Let me explain what I mean by the term "questionable." When I say that a practice is questionable, I am not saying that the doctor is either incompetent, outdated, or dishonest. Rather, I am saying, based on what I have either read or experienced, that a specific practice should be questioned or doubted. Until the data can give you a satisfactory explanation that you can verify, either through other professional opinions or supported by additional research, be careful.

Below I will describe the questionable practice and then explain why I believe it to be so.

Questionable Practice: As a result of the advent of the nerve-sparing radical prostatectomy technique, many urologists are overemphasizing the preservation of potency and are leaving some patients with persistent local disease, as indicated by a research study by Drs. Mark Rosen, Peter Scandino, et al., of Baylor College of Medicine in Houston, Texas.

Reason: This study reports that Stage A and B cancer patients who had a radical prostatectomy continue to have residual cancer outside the prostate gland. The report goes on to state that some of the patients with extraprostatic tumor might have been cured if the urologist had also removed the neurovascular bundle in addition to the prostate gland and the seminal vesicles.

All physicians who are going to operate on a patient for prostate cancer, even though they will use the nerve-sparing surgical technique, should warn their patients that if the disease has spread further than what they had suspected, they may have to abandon the procedure in order to get all of the cancer. I also understand that if the gland is unusually enlarged, doctors may not be able to save the nerves if they intend to cure the disease. This, too, should be brought to the attention of patients.

Questionable Practice: Some radiation oncologists recommend to their prostate cancer patients who are seventy and over to just wait and see without definite guidelines.

Reason: With some older patients, watchful waiting may be an appropriate approach. However, before no treatment can or should be an acceptable decision, the urologist should establish a wait-and-see criteria, such as the following:

- PSA level: less than 10.0 ng/ml
- Stage: A or B
- Age: Seventy years and older
- Type of tumor: Well-differentiated
- Gleason score: 4 or less

- Cancer cells characteristics: Diploid
- Other tests: Negative CT scan, MRI, and bone scan

Once a watchful waiting criteria is established, it should be the basis for wait-and-see patients. Even with this criteria, there is no guarantee that the patient's cancer will remain dormant. In any case, the urologist should have a contingency plan in place if the cancer happens to "take off." Such a plan should include combination hormonal therapy. One of my reviewers maintains that PSA level and stage migration are two indicators he uses as a criterion for watchful waiting patients.

Questionable Practice: Some doctors still rely solely on the digital rectal examination alone to detect cancer of the prostate.

Reason: The digital rectal examination alone is insufficient to detect cancer of the prostate. The digital rectal examination plus the PSA blood test will enable the physician to diagnose a higher number of men with prostate cancer. Research seems to indicate that the digital rectal examination alone only detects less than 20 percent of men with prostate cancer, while the digital rectal examination plus the PSA blood test are able to detect prostate cancer at the rate of slightly more than 60 percent. As stated before, every African-American male 40 and over and every white male 50 and over should demand that their doctors give them the digital rectal examination and the PSA blood test.

Questionable Practice: Based on conversations with several prostate cancer patients, a few doctors continue to give their patients estrogen without considering the new hormone drugs or the serious side effects of estrogen.

Reason: Estrogen tablets have been shown to have adverse side effects on the heart and major blood vessels and can quite possibly cause cardiovascular complications in the patient. From 1961 to 1980, when Charles Huggins, M.D., of the Ben May Institute of the University of Chicago, Illinois, and his colleagues published their study on the role of androgens of testicular origin in prostate cancer, the standard treatment for advanced prostate cancer was surgical castration or the blocking of androgen by the testes with high doses of estrogen. However, these two approaches proved to be temporary responses in 60 to 80 percent of the patients. Following the start of treatment, 20 to 40 percent of the patients did not show any improvement in the disease. In addition, 50 percent who initially responded to the treatment showed a recurrence of the cancer within one year. Furthermore, when relapse of the cancer occurred, the prognosis was poor and 50 percent of the patients were expected to die within 6 months.

Questionable Practice: Some doctors delay giving combination hormonal therapy to their Stage D prostate cancer patients until they develop symptoms of bone pain.

Reason: Extensive studies conducted by Crawford, et.al., National Cancer Institute International Group study, EORTC 30 852, and Dr. Labrie, proved that the earlier prostate cancer patients (whose cancer had spread to other organs in their bodies) are administered combination hormonal treatment, the longer is their life expectancy. These studies proved that patients with 1 to 5 bone lesions have a median time of survival in excess of 8 years. Those who have from 6 to 10 bone lesions reduced that median time of survival to 3.56 years.

This proves that doctors who recommend to their patients postponement of combination hormonal treatment until the symptoms are evident or until they experience pain is due to their lack of awareness of the research. Since combination hormonal treatment usually will not cause any harm to the body, other than some mild side effects, it is unbelievable that a doctor will wait before doing anything. After all, a man's life is in jeopardy.

Questionable Practice: Very few prostate cancer patients have either received or even heard of a DNA ploidy analysis. PAACT's *Cancer Communication* (December 1992) indicates that only 5 percent of patients have had this study performed.

Reason: DNA ploidy analysis by flow cytometry can be an extremely valuable study to assess prostate cancer tissue characteristics. Of those studied, 71 percent of patients had diploid characteristics, that is, cancer cells that are slow growing and less likely to spread through the body. As a result, many of these patients will not die of prostate cancer, but from some other disease. Some of these men will be ideal candidates for watchful waiting.

Questionable Practice: Many of the patients at one of my prostate cancer support groups maintained that even though they had enlarged prostates, their physicians failed to put them on combination hormonal therapy to debulk their prostates and make them more manageable for treatment.

Answer: Physicians have known for some time that the smaller the prostate gland, the easier it is to treat it. Why some doctors fail to shrink their patients' prostates prior to treatment puzzles me. I personally recommend all patients with an enlarged prostate to request that their doctors put them on combination hormonal therapy to shrink their prostate prior to the primary treatment (unless the disease is in the very early stages), regardless if the treatment is radical prostatectomy, external beam radiation, cryosurgery, seed implantation, etc.

Questionable Practice: Most doctors tend to be conservative, and are reluctant to recommend to their patients nontraditional treatments for prostate cancer, such as cryosurgery, seed implantation, hyperthermia, et.al., because there are no five- and ten-year-old statistical survival studies.

Reason: Let us take cryosurgery as an example. Some patients who had traditional treatments for prostate cancer, such as radical prostatectomy or external beam radiation, have had a recurrence of the cancer. If a patient has thoroughly studied all the traditional and nontraditional treatments for prostate cancer and has opted for cryosurgery, his urologist should strongly support him, since the side effects for cryosurgery seem to be more tolerable than those of a radical prostat tomy. This treatment also has a lower risk of morbidity or damaging side effects than either radical prostatectomy or external beam radiation. Cryosurgery appears to be one nontraditional treatment that deserves some consideration. After all, if a nontraditional treatment is a patient's final option, he may be able to use a traditional treatment as a back up. I see nothing wrong with this reasoning, particularly because cryosurgery is being used as a primary treatment and has been performed on patients who have had a recurrence of the disease using traditional treatments. In addition, if the first freezing does not rid the patient of all the disease, it can be repeated in order to do so.

Questionable Practice: Some doctors fail to properly follow up in a timely manner on their patients who have elevated PSA levels. Even when they do, it is usually one year after the initial PSA. As a result, the disease in most cases has spread.

Reason: Several physicians have informed me that the only procedure when a patient has an elevated PSA is to recheck it in three to four months. My urologists stated that even if they have not found any traces of cancer in the prostate, they will request their patients to reappear in their offices in three months for a new digital rectal examination and PSA blood test. Even if these visits proved negative, they would require their patients to come back for another blood test and a biopsy in three months.

As stated previously, I believe that when a urologist is performing the biopsy, a minimum of six (technically known as sextant biopsy) punctures should be performed. My reason for saying this is that minute cancer cells may be in the prostate gland and unless several punctures are made to detect these, a patient may have cancer of the prostate that may go undetected for years.

Questionable Practice: Research seems to suggest that numerous doctors tend to "understage" their prostate cancer patient when making a diagnosis. It is not uncommon for patients to be diagnosed as Stage A or B, only to discover during surgery that the patient was actually at Stage D, and the operation did not proceed.

Reason: Even though doctors may use a variety of tests to arrive at a stage for their patients with prostate cancer, the best way to determine a person's stage is when the prostate gland is surgically removed. At this time, the pathologist can identify the tumor and examine the tissues under a microscope with a technique known as whole mount evaluation. The doctor can determine the patient's true stage by testing these slices throughout the entire specimen, including the unsuspected cancers unrelated to the tumor that has already been detected. Thomas Stamey, M.D., et al., of Stanford University in Stanford, California maintained that when the whole mount evaluation was conducted, more malignant tumors were found than the tumor that was initially detected. A study published by Drs. Robert Donohue and Gary Miller of the University of Colorado in Denver, Colorado, also supports the finding by Dr. Stamey by locating additional tumors beyond the prostate gland in a majority of patients. These studies proved that patients who are identified as being at either Stage A or B are at times really pathologically at Stage C.

I therefore suggest that an improved method be developed to determine a patient's stage, other than the various tests currently used, that is, as accurate as the whole mount evaluation. What it is, I do not know. It is up to the medical profession to find an improved way to stage a person with prostate cancer rather than to guess.

Questionable Practice: Quite often, patients who are being diagnosed for treatment are left in limbo; that is, nothing is being done about their cancer until a full diagnosis has been made.

Reason: The research is clear: Combination hormonal therapy is strongly recommended for patients with prostate cancer, with the exception of early-staged patients, regardless of the treatment. Doesn't it make sense to slow down the growth of cancer prior to treatment? It will not harm patients, and in many instances, it will prove to be very beneficial.

Questionable Practice: Some Stage D patients are refusing their doctors' recommendations for treatment of prostate cancer and are instead requesting combination hormonal therapy treatment only to be denied the treatment by their doctors (*Cancer Communication*, May 1993).

Reason: The basis for these doctors' refusal was that flutamide, which is used to block androgen at the receptor sites of the prostate cancer cells, was not necessary and had no proven positive results in the treatment of prostate cancer. Research that proved to the contrary has led to lawsuits being brought against some doctors for malpractice. Dr. E. David Crawford, et.al., conducted a controlled trial of luprolide with and without flutamide in prostatic carcinoma, and settled this question as early as 1989 (*New England Journal of Medicine*, 321:418-424, August 17, 1989) by saying, "We conclude that in patients with advanced prostate cancer, treatment with luprolide and flutamide is superior to treatment with luprolide alone." However, one of my reviewers maintains that this is not true. He stated that there is relatively no difference with poor performance status patients.

Questionable Practice: Some doctors fail to do their homework to remain abreast of current research and findings, and as a result, they present incorrect or inaccurate information to patients suffering from prostate cancer.

Reason: There is no excuse for a urologist to tell his patient, for example, that the upper control limit of the PSA test is 7.0 ng/ml when it is 4.0 ng/ml or to perform a biopsy without an ultrasound probe. There is no justifiable reason for this. Just review some of the comments published in a few editions of PAACT's *Cancer Communication* newsletter:

J.P., Beaverton, OR:

Last year at this time, we [the patient and his wife] were told that as his cancer spreads "we will radiate." Those words are burned into my brain: "Why let it spread?" With combination therapy it won't—at least not in his case. We had to fight every step of the way, from uninformed doctors, doctors who scoffed at combination therapy, to doctors who felt it was "not fair to the insurance company to pay for it."

Listen to what one physician has to say about this questionable practice:

You make a point over and over again of apparent wide-spread medical malpractice in regard to the diagnosis and treatment of prostate cancer. In my experience, this is true and in fact, I myself may have fallen into that category of which your newsletter speaks in the past, not because of greed as you indicate may be the case of many physicians (especially the surgeons—which I am not) but rather due to ignorance. Everyday I and my colleagues see a number of types of patients and it is impossible to be familiar with all of the latest treatment methods for each of the various conditions that the patient comes to the doctor for. The very fact that the PAACT newsletter exists speaks to the truth of this fact. As a practicing physician, it is extremely difficult to keep up on even one small area of research much less thousands. Another problem is remembering all of the facts needed at the time of the office visit in order to provide the optimum care. The information may be in a journal on my desk at home or in my library but finding information needed at the particular time that it is needed is generally impossible. In regards to the latest information on prostate cancer—that information will not generally be available to me since it is information given at meetings that I have not been invited to or could not attend. Therefore this information can only reach me by way of the PAACT newsletter since I know of no other newsletter that reviews these findings.

I will close by saying that in my opinion, until every doctor in this country who treats men over the age of 40 has this type of information on his or her desk, you will continue to see the "medical ignorance" syndrome and this will continue to cause the needless pain, suffering, and death of thousands of men.

W.S., Jamestown, New York:

Early in 1992 my oncologist put me on Emcyt, and results were "so." In a few months, my PSA had climbed
from 44 to 85.

Then I came across your article in the September *Cancer
Communication* newsletter that recommended it be sup-
plemented with Velban. I showed the article to my oncologist and he went along with it. I have finished two
cycles of treatment (six weeks on both drugs, then two
weeks off represents one cycle). Almost immediately I
had felt a lot better, and my latest PSA was back down
to the forties.

The following is a letter cited in PAACT's *Cancer Communication* newsletter and a response to that letter:

J.M., Williamsburg, Virginia:

Permit me to make a few comments. I feel my oncologist, being a professional in the health field, will want
to know the source of your writings. It is not clear
whether the writer is paraphrasing from the source, or
whether he is simply giving his own views, or express-
ing something he has previously learned from one or
more other sources.

For example, you write convincingly that flutamide
should be taken every eight hours, not just "three times
daily." Neither my urologist nor oncologist has ever
mentioned this regimen. I would feel much more secure
if I could give him the source for his advice, as I am sure
he will feel defensive because he didn't give the advice
himself.

Editor: Thanks for responding with your letter regarding the materials supplied by our organization. Accept-

ing criticism is not easy for most of us, although much of what you say is well founded. Between sending you the initial information and receiving your letter, we completed revising some of our materials, which now include several reference notations.

We do not intend for anyone to simply "take our word" without thoughtful questioning. Mr. Ney has spent the past eight to nine years concentrating on research and interactive discussion with a large number of reputable research physicians, recognized as authorities on prostate cancer. It is not possible for any one individual to know everything there is about any one topic, although when one has the opportunity to study only one topic for a number of years, one can gain an extensive understanding. Over the years, Mr. Ney has come to be recognized as an authority in his own right. The knowledge that he has gained, and the information that we are able to share through the network of the PAACT organization is directed from the patient's standpoint.

The thrust of patient advocacy is to enable the patient to be in control of the management of his own illness. We hope to instill in you the desire to know as much as you can learn about what will certainly affect the rest of your life. It is surely not to be assumed that a physician should be excluded from the care of the patient, but an appropriate role must be assumed by joint participation. It is your life that is at stake. It is a crucial mistake to take for granted that your physician will always know what is best for you.

Quite frankly, if anything we say or anything you say to your physician causes him or her to feel defensive, then you have a pretty reliable indicator that the physician may be more concerned with his or her own interests than your well being. To use your example, the product information for Eulexin, supplied by the pharmaceutical company to all physicians who prescribe the medication and published annually in the *Physician's Desk Reference*, clearly indicates that the drug is to be prescribed at eight to nine hour intervals. Would you consider the developer and manufacturer of the drug to be an adequate authority on the issue of every eight-hour dosing? Sadly, it seems that the majority of physicians often do not make the effort to fully understand the medications they prescribe. Could that be why neither your urologist nor your oncologist has ever mentioned this regimen?

Do not misunderstand my questions. I do not mean to imply that your physicians are incompetent. You have to determine, however, how to make them accountable to *you* to ensure that you receive the absolute best possible care. It seems that we only have one opportunity at life, at least in the human form that we know. Most of us would like to protect it as carefully as we can.

B.N., St. Peter, Missouri:

Dear Sirs:

While talking with you about 6 weeks ago, you recommended the use of cytadren and hydrocortisone. At that time, I had passed the chemotherapy trials and was taking nothing. I was almost unable to walk, and the quality of life was absolutely zero.

Now I am walking about 3/4 of a mile, the swelling has receded some in my thighs and ankles, and the quality of life is almost normal. My PSA level has gone from 82 to 52.

Questionable Practice: Some doctors fail to properly communicate to their prostate cancer patients and demonstrate insensitivity toward them.

Reason: Similar to the last questionable practice, there is absolutely no justifiable reason for doctors to fail to communicate to their patients. Neither is there an adequate reason for them to demonstrate insensitivity.

Let us review some of the comments cited in PAACT's *Cancer Communication* newsletter:

Comments from an attorney:

> I am an attorney and one who had a radical prostatectomy for prostate cancer in January 1987. I, too, have a horror story. Thus, I believe I am qualified to offer you some suggestions...

> Having gone through the experience I did, I keep trying to understand how such a thing could happen in today's world and why I feel so outraged. The essence of the problem is the special relationship of truth and confidence which doctors have with their patients. There are numerous different types of trust relationships, but they all arise when one person holds himself out to others as having special knowledge, skill, or ability to come to him or her with their particular problem in their area of expertise. Thus, an attorney-client, accountant-client, dentist-patient, etc., are all examples of a trust relationship. In view of the difference in the understanding between the two persons in the trust relationship, the law (equity and good conscience) attempts to balance the playing field. Thus, it requires the trustee (doctors) to have fair and honorable dealings with the patient. A subset of this requirement is that the trustee has a duty to make a full and meaningful disclosure of all material facts to the patient-beneficiary concerning the matter entrusted to the trustee. Note that this is a significantly different relationship than

that involved where a person is buying a used car. The used car salesman is expected to tout his wares using superlatives and half-truths. Prior to the recent consumer protection laws, the only duty imposed on the used car salesman was not to make an intentional misrepresentation of a material fact, i.e., commit fraud or deceit. Doctors should be held to a higher standard than used car salesmen.

An intentional, consented touching or contact with another person constitutes battery, a civil wrong for which the law provides damages. Certainly, a radical prostatectomy or other invasive medical procedures constitute such a battery unless the patient gives consent. However, one cannot consent to that which he does not understand, at least in a broad, general sense. Thus, the law requires the patient to give his "informed consent." The concept of informed consent related back to the trust principle which requires the trustee to make a full and meaningful disclosure to the beneficiary.

The fact is that too many persons hold themselves out to the world as "doctors" but deal with their patients as though they were used car salesman. A friend of mine has told me, "You've got to be smart enough to protect yourself against them."But a patient expects that his doctor is on his side to provide for his best interest rather than a used car salesman against whom he has to protect his own best interest. Thus, some doctors do not have fair and honorable dealings with their patients but engage in withholding material facts, telling half-truths, communicating in medical jargon which does not make a meaningful disclosure to the patient in a way he can understand, and in some cases, actively or passively withholding important, material information from the patient. A patient facing cancer is very vulnerable and is anxious to place his or her trust in a doctor, even though such trust may be misplaced.

The doctors in Oregon have caused the Oregon legislature to enact a law requiring the patient to make a request for a more detailed explanation of the procedure or treatment after the doctor makes only a general explanation (ORS 677.097). Thus, the doctors' common law duty to make a full and meaningful disclosure has been modified by statute. However, the pragmatic basis for the common law trust rule still exists. In my case, after only one meeting at which a radical prostatectomy was recommended, the doctor refused to see me a second time before the surgery. Apparently, his conscience was clear that he had fulfilled his statutory duty by using his medical jargon which no layman could understand in one setting.

Thus, as explained above, the problem as I see it rests with the doctor's very important obligation to make a full and meaningful disclosure of all material facts including alternative procedures to the patient. I believe there are many doctors who do not fulfill this responsibility. Thus, the root cause of many of the medical horror stories you refer to lies in two areas: 1) lack of compassion for a hurting patient, and 2) lack of a meaningful communication by the doctor to the patient as to the course of action and possible alternative courses of action. As you no doubt know, there are a host of explanations offered by doctors in support of their conduct. However, your 60,000 horror stories demonstrate that these explanations fail to satisfy the patient's "need to know."

Of course, the competency of the doctor raises additional issues. The plain and simple truth is that the medical profession does not adequately police its doctors to weed out the ones who are incompetent or to rebuke those who engage in substandard practices. As a consequence, the entire medical profession must suffer for the sins of a few.

R.R., Bloomington, Indiana:

I am amazed at the professional *ignorance* and *indifference* by urologists, radiation oncologists, and doctors about treating prostate cancer. I will tell you this—I intend to fight for the right to live and do not intend to take as gospel the word of some doctors...information that they cannot back up with medical facts.

As an example, the 35 radiation treatments that they gave me that may or may not have been necessary and then later have my urologist tell me of all the harmful side effects *after* I had taken the treatments. I want facts and will continue to ask questions until I get answers backed up by medical research and not doctor mumbojumbo.

[The above letters all come from PAACT. You are probably wondering why I devoted so much attention to this organization. The answer is simply because PAACT is your organization. Even if you are not a member, you are entitled to all the benefits accorded to members. Numerous letters are sent in to the main office by prostate cancer victims conveying the results of their knowledge and experiences that are communicated to members and nonmembers via PAACT's newsletter. Some readers may not agree. I think by recounting these letters and comments, others can benefit. In fact, who knows, these comments may save lives or at least improve the quality of life for those patients with metastasized prostate cancer.]

Questionable Practice: Recently I attended a prostate cancer support subgroup of men who had undergone radical prostatectomies. I queried the participants and asked if their doctors had ever discussed with them the need to preserve and store their tissues should there be a recurrence of the disease. Not to my surprise, not one of the twenty-two men indicated affirmatively. In fact, several of the men became annoyed and lambasted doctors in general.

Reason: When a radical prostatectomy—or any surgical procedure for that matter—results in the removal of a diseased tissue, the patient's tissues should be stored and preserved. If there should be a recurrence of the cancer, the tissue could be used for a chemosensitivity study that would be able to indicate the best method for further treatment. In addition, there are several research studies underway using the patient's own tissue for the development of a vaccine for the treatment of prostate cancer. The tissues that are removed from your body are your property. Even if your urologist or cancer surgeon does not mention the preservation of your tissue, you have every right to do so. However, one of my reviewers maintains that much needs to be done and perhaps in the future, we may have monoclonal antibodies that will allow us to carry out this feat.

Questionable Practice: Sometimes doctors fail to be creative in recommending various treatments for prostate cancer to their patients.

Reason: Most doctors tend to be sold totally on the traditional techniques for treating prostate cancer; that is, they think conservatively and thus may not be recommending to their patients the best treatments for their disease. First, let us consider a traditional treatment for prostate cancer. Wouldn't it be more advantageous for the patients if the doctor were to recommend ultrasound transrectal brachytherapy followed by external beam radiation rather than merely external beam radiation? Usually when external beam radiation is the treatment of choice, it is believed that it will pick up any marginal disease. However, if ultrasound transrectal brachytherapy is used as a primary treatment, it would be an advantage over external beam radiation to destroy the bulk of the disease either through improved accuracy or increased dosages. External beam radiation could then be used to apply more rads (unit of measure for radiation) to treat any marginal disease. Now, let us consider a nontraditional treatment for prostate cancer. Let us say that a patient refused the doctor's recommendation of external beam radiation and opted for cryosurgery. Isn't it possible for the patient to receive external beam radiation therapy or a repeat of cryosurgery if the initial cryosurgery treatment failed to successfully destroy all of the cancer?

Questionable Practice: Even though the digital rectal examination is only one means to detect prostate cancer in patients, far too many doctors fail to perform this procedure, which may be the reason why many men who are diagnosed with prostate cancer are detected after the "cure period" and suffer from metastatic prostate cancer.

Reason: The Cleveland Clinic *Journal of Medicine* (Vol. 59, No. 4, P. 386) verified this questionable practice when it found that in a survey of 433 men over the age of 40 performed at the Cleveland Clinic in 1989 and 1990, 67 percent said they had not had a digital rectal examination performed in the previous year. More alarming was that of the 153 men who did report having a general physical examination in the previous year, the digital rectal examination was included only 56 percent of the time.

Questionable Practice: A gold standard for prostate cancer is reported to be radical prostatectomy. And the gold standard for removing testosterone from the body of the human male is bilateral orchiectomy, or surgical removal of both of the testes.

Reason: I question whether these standards are valid when you consider that many physicians are practicing new treatments and advancements in medical technology. I also feel the term gold standard needs to be redefined. Today, for example, combination hormonal therapy is sometimes given as a preliminary treatment to debulk and downstage the prostate cancer to make the tumor more manageable for treatment. Sometimes after the operation, external beam radiation is given in order to treat any marginal disease. As a result of the transrectal ultrasound machine, treatments that were once unsuccessful, such as those associated with brachytherapy, are becoming more successful in killing cancerous cells in the prostate.

The old definition of gold standard, which addresses only one treatment, should be revised to include any preliminary and/or salvage treatment, as well as any specific medical technology. After all, whatever success is realized through radical prostatectomy would also be due to any preliminary treatment and/or salvage treatment, as well as the medical technology. In essence, the new definition would define a "process" made up of several components or parts. If any component is omitted, the entire process (treatment) would be adversely affected.

I have not been able to ascertain the current definition of gold standard from my research and studies. However, I would redefine gold standard (the process) as follows:

One or a combination of treatments for prostate cancer which have proven to be effective through research and studies that have maximized the number of patients surviving the disease with minimal side effects over a ten-year period. The medical technology used to deliver any radiation should have a three-dimensional imaging capacity.

As a result, I would revise the two gold standards cited above using my definition of gold standards as follows:

The administration of six months of combination hormonal therapy as a preliminary treatment to make an enlarged prostate more manageable for treatment followed by radical prostatectomy. In some cases, external beam radiation may be used as a salvage treatment to eliminate any marginal disease.

Many urologists are shifting from a single treatment (radical prostatectomy) for prostate cancer to a multiple treatment approach (combination hormonal treatment if the patient has an enlarged prostate and external beam radiation if there is suspicion of marginal disease) to enhance their cure rate. Studies and experience seem to be leading to the following as a gold standard using my definition:

> The administration of six months of combination hormonal therapy to debulk and downstage an enlarged tumor followed by internal radiation using a three-dimensional computer image with transrectal ultrasound technology. Sometimes a modest dose of external beam radiation is used prior to seed implantation to eliminate any marginal disease.

Notice that my definition actually includes the identification of technology to be used in the treatment process. This is because with different technology, you are likely to get different treatment results. If nothing else, this questionable practice should stir some debate over the current antiquated gold standard definition.

Questionable Practice: Unfortunately, many medical specialty boards permit "grandfathering" whereby already-certified doctors do not have to be recertified and recertification requirements apply only to newly-certified doctors.

Reason: This is perhaps one of the most ridiculous policies I came across during my studies and readings. The doctors who perhaps need to update their studies and practices the most are not required to do so. No wonder that tens of thousands of doctors are being sued for malpractice annually. It appears that specialty boards are more concerned about appeasing their membership than protecting patients against outmoded doctors. However, I do not blame the board entirely, a few states must take some of the blame. One such state is New York. A few years ago the Medical Society of New York State required of its members a minimum number of continuing education credits over a three-year period, however, because the State of New York did not require any credits, the society dropped its requirements.

No doubt there are countless other questionable practices that should be considered. The problem for you is to fortify yourself with as much knowledge and research about prostate cancer as is humanly possible, and look for differences of opinions. Use your wisdom to the best of your ability to make sound decisions regarding the diagnosis, treatment, and prognosis of prostate cancer.

CHAPTER FOUR

What I Did to Gain Support and Acquire Knowledge About My Condition

In a study of 86 women with breast cancer, David Spiegel, M.D., professor of psychiatry at Stanford University School of Medicine, discovered that women who participated in weekly support group sessions lived an average of 18 months longer than those who did not. In fact, the study also revealed that the more frequently a woman attended these sessions, the greater her benefits. For example, the average survival time for women who attended between 1 and 10 support group sessions was 36.2 months. This figure jumped to 41.5 months for women who attended more than 10 sessions.

Although I have not been able to find a similar study for men with prostate cancer, I believe that participation in prostate cancer support groups should extend the longevity of men also. I also feel that support groups have a positive effect on a patient's psychological behavior by providing a buffer against stress and anxiety, thereby cushioning the body from the consequences of stress hormones. As a result, the body's immune system is able to counteract the effects of prostate cancer more efficiently.

Living with prostate cancer will be difficult for you as well as for those who care for you. Everyone involved faces a multitude of problems, challenges, and decisions. It is easier to deal with those difficulties when people with similar needs get together to share information and support each other. Emotional support is equally important, because you begin to realize that you are not alone with your problems.

Togetherness can prove to be most comforting. Basically, support groups are self-help organizations made up of patients afflicted with a similar disease. Assistance is provided to these groups on a continuous basis and they are usually led by a social worker. Sometimes they are led by physicians or nurses. I joined three support groups: two groups where I actually attended monthly meetings, and additional groups that I refer to as education groups. One of these was to receive its monthly newsletter, and the other, to become familiar with all its varied services.

The first support group I joined was affiliated with the Maimonides Hospital in Brooklyn, New York. Membership in this support group varies from meeting to meeting, but at no time does it consist of more than two dozen members. Brooklyn is a very large area, so I was astounded when I first saw the limited number of participants. However, with time, I began to like the small size of the group. Carol Becker was the social worker who moderated the meetings and led the group meeting. The meetings usually began with new members introducing themselves and indicating where they were in the diagnosis and/or treatment of their disease. Using the language of the field, new members were asked questions pertaining to their PSA level, Gleason score, stage, etc. Usually, these terms meant nothing to most newcomers, thus beginning their education and supportive process.

We tended to be sensitive to a new member's need for information, and offered advice when we felt it was warranted. Such an example occurred in a recent meeting when a newcomer told us his doctor had recommended estrogen. I quickly told him the side effects of this drug and asked him to consider seeking a doctor who is more current in the treatment of cancer. I further elaborated on other more manageable hormones.

This is what one does in support group meetings. We give a great deal of our own personal experience as well as listen to others to learn something new. A person coming into our group had better know his PSA level, Gleason score, stage, etc. If not, he will be overwhelmed by the language. Recently, a new member who had just received a radical prostatectomy was astounded when he could not respond to the group's queries regarding his PSA level and Gleason score.

I also attend an US TOO International, Inc., prostate cancer support group at the Memorial Sloan-Kettering Cancer Research Center because it has a much larger number of participants than the Brooklyn support group. About 150 men and women attend these monthly sessions. Several professional people are usually there to answer any questions posed by the participants. At the beginning of the support group session, a brief presentation is made regarding a subject of interest to members. After this presentation, the group is divided into several smaller groups. A leader is designated to lead these smaller groups based on what treatment he chose. These small sessions are usually identified as a stage A and B group, stage C and D group, and a wives' group. In these sessions, the leader begins by telling something about his treatment and the rest of the group members join in by using a comment from the leader or a member as a springboard to relate information about his own individual diagnoses and treatments. The meetings are very informative due to the number of attendees in each group and the wide range of experiences.

US TOO is about four years old. It has 225 groups in 47 states, including Washington, D.C.; 4 provinces in Canada, and Istanbul, Turkey. Edward C. Kaps is co-founder of US TOO. Between the American Foundation for Urologic Disease, Inc., and US TOO, an average of more than 2,500 telephone calls are made to its office in Scottsdale, Arizona. John M. Moenck is editor-in-chief of its newsletter. Each monthly issue contains a wealth of information, such as the following:

- Highly interesting articles by physicians and other professionals in areas of interest and value to men (and their families and friends) who were diagnosed and/or treated for prostate cancer.

- Information, ideas, suggestions, and help regarding diagnosis and treatment; what US TOO groups are doing for programs; outreach into their communities. Anything pertinent is welcome and encouraged to be submitted to the managing editor for publication consideration.

- Questions—with appropriate answers or comments by appropriate persons—relating to anything about prostate cancer, symptoms, diagnosis, treatment, patient care in the hospital and at home; and helpful ideas for the caregiver (spouse, significant other, family member, or other person).

- Letters to the Editor (readers have the opportunity to comment on anything relating in any way to prostate cancer).

- "What's Happening...?" (a summation, a distillation of news and information taken from the newsletters of US TOO groups—what special programs or program ideas groups are having, events group members are participating in, community publicity, screenings, informationals, and publicity accomplishments, anything that will be of interest, value, and help to other US TOO groups).

- Photographs that illustrate points or show something outstanding or unusual or enhance an idea or story.

- "How I (We) Handled It" (how prostate cancer survivors and their caregivers have dealt with different situations and problems, relating to incontinence, impotence, sex, eating, sleeping, nutrition, pain control, comfort in the hospital and at home; how to be an appreciative patient from the patient's point of view).

- "Caring for the Caregiver" (helping the caregiver to keep his or her balance, sense of humor; things for the caregiver to do, by him or herself and/or with others).

- Cancer resources (books, brochures, videotapes, films, support groups; names, addresses, and phone numbers of helpful resources).

The Medical Advisory and Contributing Editors Board of US TOO includes the members of the Prostate Health Council of the American Foundation for Urologic Disease.

An article in a recent edition of the US TOO newsletter included an article in which one of the founders of the organization who had a PSA level over 4,000 ng/ml said he felt the need to initiate a separate high-risers US TOO prostate cancer support group to give special help and support to those prostate cancer patients whose disease has spread beyond the prostate. A high-riser includes the following:

1) An individual whose PSA rises more than .75 ng/ml.

2) An individual with a detectable PSA following radical prostatectomy.

3) An individual whose PSA is not reduced following radiation therapy.

4) An individual who has a positive bone scan, CT scan, X-ray, or MRI, regardless of PSA.

5) any other individual with a PSA above 10 ng/ml.

Although the two support groups and the subscription to US TOO International newsletter proved to be beneficial for expanding my knowledge about prostate cancer, most of my knowledge was gained as a result of joining PAACT. This non-profit organization is the largest prostate cancer affiliation in the world. It is led by a champion, Lloyd Ney, who looked death squarely in the eye in 1982 when he had 32 cancer lesions throughout his skeleton. His doctor gave him a maximum of six months to live. Using a combination of luprolide and flutamide, Mr. Ney is alive today without a trace of prostate cancer.

When Ney found out he had cancer, he did not pity himself, nor did he give up. Instead, he became stubborn, as champions are. He was going to beat this terrible disease using knowledge and information as his weapons. Today, PAACT, is a symbol of life and hope for millions of men who have prostate cancer. Look at the numerous activities PAACT has achieved for its members and nonmembers, to say the least.

PAACT recognized the significant contribution of PSA level, recommending its use as early as 1989 for a more accurate diagnosis of prostate cancer and as a monitoring biomarker of activity and progression. In 1984, PAACT was formed based on the prediction that combination hormonal therapy should be the first choice of treatment for prostate cancer (and still, there are physicians who refuse to take heed). Medications such as luprolide and flutamide are very expensive; however, members of PAACT can call toll-free at 1-800-227-1195 to receive their prescriptions at substantial savings.

Since its inception, PAACT has conducted extensive research and investigations, and has shared the results of its efforts with both patients and physicians. One of the primary objectives of PAACT is to educate the patient so he is aware of all of the prostate cancer treatment option available to him. As a result, this enables him to exert his right to select his preferential treatment based on his informed judgement.

PAACT has also established an information electronic mailbox that is available twenty-four hours a day, seven days per week, and can be used to respond to your request for information on a variety of diagnostic and treatment options. Just dial (616) 453-1351, select your subject matter from the subjects below, and dial the access number. What is good about this service is that you do not have to be a member of PAACT to have access to this electronic mailbox.

Early in my quest for knowledge, I used this service at least six times. I also have informed perhaps three or four dozen others about the availability of the PAACT electronic mailbox. Go ahead, select subject matter. Start off with access number three and listen to the general information about PAACT and prostate cancer. Get a notepad ready before you dial and jot down information that is pertinent to you. Figure 4.1 identifies information available through PAACT's new electronic message mailbox.

PAACT has dedicated space in its *Cancer Communication* newsletter in an effort to enable its members to stay abreast of the latest techniques, products, and medical briefs.

Each year, PAACT disseminates a questionnaire on some aspect of prostate cancer to its 17,000 members. Members are asked to take a few minutes to complete the form and return it as soon as possible. PAACT publishes the results.

PAACT has established a Prostate Tumor Tissue Bank to store a portion of member's tumor tissue following surgery or biopsy. These tissues may be useful for discovering a vaccine for prostate cancer in the future. Studies at the National Cancer Institute and Memorial Sloan-Kettering Cancer Research Center have shown responses to vaccines containing gene inserts. These types of vaccines may prove useful in the treatment of prostate cancer that has spread beyond the gland.

PAACT is accumulating materials for a book to be entitled, *Prostate Cancer and Medical Felony: A Chronicle of Humor, Human Interest, and Horror.* The book will be comprised of excerpts selected from more than 60,000 letters received since its inception from prostate cancer patients, wives, widows, and families. When the book is published, the net proceeds will go to the PAACT Cancer Foundation Fund. This book will present the general audience with problems of medical practice in the diagnosis and treatment of patients with advanced prostate cancer.

A strong point of PAACT is that it strives to remain abreast of new developments in the detection, diagnosis, evaluation, and treatment for prostate cancer in all stages. New developments come across the staff desk almost daily. However, before its members receive this information through either the electronic mailbox, the *Cancer Communication* newsletter, or the telephone, these developments are thoroughly researched and investigated.

Figure 4.1
Information Available on PAACT's Electronic Mailbox

Access No.	Time Length (min., secs.)	Subject
1#	1:55	Introduction to Listening Options and Menu Choices
2#	2:23	Treatment of Hormone Refractory Disease
3#	2:59	General Information About PAACT and Prostate Cancer
4#	1:13	Tumor Necrosis Treatment (TNT Monoclonal Antibody)
5#	1:16	Prostatis and Benign Prostatic Hyperplasia
6#	1:41	PSA # (Prostate Specific Antigen)
7#	3:38	DNA Ploidy Analysis: "To Treat, or Not to Treat"
8#	2:34	Down-Voluming/Downstaging with Combination Therapy
9#		[currently unused]
10#	1:38	Pain Management
11#		[currently unused]
12#	2:23	The Importance of Transrectal Ultrasound (TRU/S) and Fine Needle Biopsy
13#	11:55	Cryosurgery: A Personal Experience

PAACT was instrumental in securing the approval of Eulexin (flutamide) in the United States and pioneered the acceptance of combination hormonal therapy. PAACT continues to stay in touch with the FDA to secure the controlled release of changes approved by foreign countries. Each year, PAACT updates its "Prostate Cancer Report," a comprehensive report on what is believed to be the most accurate and concise assimilation of data available on prostate cancer.

PAACT maintains contact and communication with many members of Congress through its chapters and members to assure that the proper attention and consideration be given to the concerns of the prostate cancer patient, and that investigative procedures are begun when the welfare of the prostate patient is in jeopardy. It also remains in contact with pharmaceutical companies to promote investigation of promising new drugs, aids in the proliferation of clinical trials, and promotes the approval of new therapies based on convincing clinical evidence of the efficacy of advanced medical treatments.

After more than eight years of accumulating data from its over 17,000 prostate cancer patients and experiencing the hindrances placed on the availability of new drugs in the treatment of cancer, PAACT has advocated a review by congress of the regulatory procedures of the FDA. Apparently, PAACT feels that it is time to take a closer look at the criteria and personnel used to evaluate the efficacy of new drugs, expand and broaden participation in Investigation of New Drugs (INDs) and accelerate the approval of New Drug Applications (NDAs). The regulatory procedures for the approval of new drugs by the FDA have been reviewed by the President's Cancer Panel ad hoc committee, and PAACT is proud that it was requested to give testimony before this committee in Bethesda, Maryland, at the request of the National Cancer Institute.

PAACT attempts to aid the semi-indigent in acquiring financial support so they can get medication by means of temporary IND applications and other available means through social agencies and other concerned groups. A local, state, and national campaign began in 1993 to construct a World Class Comprehensive Cancer Research Institute to serve the 2.5 million population of western Michigan, the state as a whole, and the world. One of the prime objectives is to provide access to new medications and clinical trials for all patients and to equip and staff the world's finest prostate cancer clinic. Through the acquisition of adequate research, personnel, and equipment, its primary objective is to use laboratory facilities to provide focus, direction, and continuity in the development of prevention, therapy, and cure of all forms of cancer. It will continue to provide education and guidance to the public at large, the patient in particular, and the medical profession as a whole.

The largest expansion of PAACT's attack on prostate cancer is the formation of PAACT-PCOG (Prostate Cancer Oncology Group), headed by E. Roy Berger, M.D., oncologist and hematologist with the North Shore Hematology/Oncology Associates in Port Jefferson Station, New York. The group is currently composed of over 100 physicians, many of whom are the leading authorities in detection, diagnosis, and treatment of prostate cancer, in the United States, Canada, and abroad, who join them to conduct privately funded clinical trials to provide better diagnostic and treatment protocols for prostate cancer.

Each year, hundreds of physicians around the United States contact PAACT for a standard of materials to update their knowledge about current trends and developments for the detection, diagnosis, evaluation, and treatment of prostate cancer. These materials consist of memorandum, guidelines, questions and answers, and factual data. Finally, PAACT engages in research from databases, medical journals, clinical trials, published and unpublished medical papers, and its own patient registry to obtain the latest and most up-to-date information on the detection, diagnosis, evaluation, and treatment of prostate cancer. The information accumulated is reviewed, published, and relayed through the organization's official newsletter, *Cancer Communication*, and other pamphlets and books.

I cannot express it too strongly. All patients afflicted with prostate cancer and physicians who desire to stay abreast of current trends, developments, and research in prostate cancer should join PAACT immediately. For patients, this one move may save or lengthen your life. For physicians, it may enable you to guide and direct patients to save their lives. If you do not believe me, read a few of the 60,000 letters that have reached PAACT's office since its inception:

A short note from M.C., a patient in Mountain View, CA:

I want to thank you for including me on PAACT's mailing list. I have prostate cancer and had a radical prostatectomy on July 31. My reason for writing you is that

I would greatly appreciate it if you would add my three older brothers, each of whom have prostate cancer, to PAACT's mailing list.

Thank you and keep up the great work.

REPLY: Do you have any other brothers? If so, they should ask to be on our mailing list, as well. The reported incidence of prostate cancer involving multiple members of a family (grandfather, father, uncles, brothers, sons) is becoming increasingly familiar. The December, 1991, issue of *The Saturday Evening Post* includes a moving article that relates to familial incidence. Those of us who have any immediate male relatives who have had prostate cancer carry a much higher risk than the general population for developing this disease.

Those of you who already have prostate cancer need to inform your uncles, brothers, sons, and nephews. They need to know that they are at risk. This is not being discussed to cause any panic, but it needs to be said, and needs to be said clearly. We need to increase awareness of the prevalence of this illness.

The PSA blood test (prostate specific antigen) makes screening for prostate cancer a very simple process, and screening is of extreme importance for male members of affected families. Through regular screening, prostate cancer, if it develops, can be detected and diagnosed at an early stage, when the potential for permanent cure would be the greatest.

Andrew D. Seidman, M.D., of Memorial Sloan-Kettering, New York, NY, writes:

I am sorry I missed you at the end of last week's PAACT-PCOG conference, but want to tell you how thoroughly I enjoyed it. I found the meeting both scientifically stimulating and educationally enlightening. You have created a unique and invaluable instrument to further the battle against prostate cancer, and I am sure the impact of the group will be significant for many patients and physicians.

In closing, I would like to admonish the National Cancer Institute because I have not found one of their publications in which it has mentioned the availability of PAACT to assist patients with prostate cancer. In some areas, PAACT is way out in front of the service that the National Cancer Institute offers. A good example is the electronic mailbox. I do not understand this, because PAACT is the largest self-help nonprofit organization for prostate cancer patients in the world.

Whenever there is a crisis, everybody needs some support. Perhaps the best self-help support involves joining local groups that are usually affiliated with local hospitals, as well as joining international support groups such as PAACT and US TOO. Although reading and researching information on prostate cancer is essential, it is perhaps more essential to join support groups to interact with other prostate cancer victims to learn and benefit from their experience. Do not make the mistake that hundreds and perhaps thousands of prostate cancer patients make. Join prostate cancer support groups prior to treatment, not after treatment. If, however, you are guilty of this deed, stay with your prostate cancer support group. Who knows? You may have a recurrence of this disease.

CHAPTER FIVE

How to Select and Communicate With Your Doctor

Several years ago the subcommittee on Oversight and Investigations of the U.S. House of Representatives reported on the surgical performance of American doctors that: "An individual may have twice the chance of dying from an operation simply by having the procedure performed at one hospital rather than another." The subcommittee indicated that the information being made available to the public concerning adequate health care was actually inadequate.

Although this report is not new, it is still true today. The quality of health care varies from one hospital to another, depending how the medical world views your doctor. If he or she is known as a competent and exacting physician who places their patients' welfare before anything else, you will get respect and maximum efficiency from the hospital staff. However, if he or she is not exacting, your doctor will not get respect or the kind of medical care their patients deserve. A doctor stated it this way: "There are two levels of care in the same hospital. The top level goes to those patients who have good doctors that demand it; the second level of care goes to those patients whose doctors are known to the hospital staff to be lazy or sloppy." So what is the meaning of the subcommittee's report?

It is saying that if you retain an excellent doctor, you will get excellent health care in your hospital.

What is a patient to do? By considering the ideas presented in this chapter, you should be able to select an excellent doctor, the most important task you can perform, and be able to effectively communicate with him or her, the second most important task.

HOW TO SELECT A DOCTOR

To select my doctor, I first obtained literature about the best doctors in the nation and chose an internist. I made an appointment to meet with him to discuss my case (my form of interviewing), at which time I reviewed his degrees and certificates and read from several of his books. I was extremely attuned to how he treated me and the rapport we had together. Once I retained my family doctor, he introduced me to one of the best doctors in New York City. The words of my internist still echo in my ears: "There are urologists and there are urologists, and I'm going to introduce you to a *urologist*."

My remaining doctors were those recommended by other excellent doctors. However, I have included in this chapter several other effective ways to select doctors that were presented to me by members of my support groups. Select one or more of the methods that you feel comfortable with.

Require either your family doctor or friends to recommend two or three names of doctors by discipline, and then prepare a list of questions in order to interview each one. (See pages 117 and 118.)

Call a department such as urology at a large hospital, and ask the secretary, "If you had to identify a doctor within the department to operate on your father, who would you recommend?" Secretaries usually know who the best doctors are in a department.

William Catalona, M.D., Chief of Urologic Surgery at George Washington University in St. Louis, Missouri, maintains that when selecting a surgeon for prostate cancer, avoid doctors who have performed fewer than 150 prostatectomies or who have patients with higher rates of incontinence and impotence than those reported in journal articles by surgeons from major hospitals. He further states, "If your surgeon cannot tell you those rates, get another doctor."

I believe it is important to go further by getting your doctor to identify several of his previous patients and for you to interview them. One of my reviewers said that he would not give this information; however, this is just what one doctor did for one of my colleagues in my Brooklyn prostate cancer support group. There is no harm in trying. In addition, query your doctor as to when he or she received training in Walsh's nerve-sparing surgical technique to preserve your potency.

My wife selected a doctor by seeing him on the television. She evaluated his knowledge of his area of expertise and sensitivity to people, mannerisms, etc. She then contacted the gynecologist via telephone and went off to Boston for her first of a number of appointments. I am not saying that you will always select an acceptable doctor in this manner; I am just providing you with an option that worked for my wife.

You can use the local medical society to give you the names of three urologists to contact and interview. Other sources that you can use to locate doctors are the State Medical Directory, the American Board of Certified Specialists, or the American Medical Association Directory, which are located in most libraries. However, I do not recommend these sources because you really do not know who you will be getting.

Collect books and magazines that list the best doctors in the nation and select from that list. For example, the October 1992 issue of *Good Housekeeping* has such a list. One recent book that deserves consideration is *Good Doctors, Bad Doctors*, by Charles B. Inlander (Viking Press, New York, 1993).

The following is a list of cancer specialists who have been reported by at least two sources to be the best in their respective areas:

Urologists:

Richard J. Ablin, Ph.D.
InnaPharma, Inc.
75 Montebello Road
Suffern, NY 10901

Dr. Samuel S. Ambrose, Jr.
Emory University Clinic
1365 Clifton Road
Atlanta, GA 30322

Dr. William H. Boyce
Bowman-Gray Medical School
300 Hawthorne Road
Winston-Salem, NC 27103

Dr. C. Eugene Carlton
Baylor College of Medicine
6560 Fannin Street
Houston, TX 77025

Dr. Roy J. Correa, Jr.
Virginia Mason Clinic
1100 Ninth Avenue
Seattle, WA 98111

Dr. George W. Drach
1501 N. Campbell Avenue
Tucson, AZ 85274

Dr. William Fair
Washington University
Medical School
One Brookings Drive
St. Louis, MO 63110

Dr. Ruben F. Gitties
Peter Bent Brigham Hospital
75 Francis Street
Boston, MA 02115

Dr. John T. Grayhack
Northwestern Memorial Hospital
707 N. Fairbanks Court
Chicago, IL 60611

Dr. Donald Griffith
Baylor College of Medicine
6560 Fannin Street
Houston, TX 70025

Dr. Thomas R. Hakala
Urological Surgery
University of Pittsburgh
Pittsburgh, PA 15213

Dr. Frank Hinman, Jr.
University of California Medical Cntr.
505 Parnassus Avenue
San Francisco, CA 94143

Dr. Joseph J. Kaufman
University of California
at Los Angeles Medical Center
10833 Leconte Avenue
Los Angeles, CA 90024

Dr. Warren Koontz
Medical College of Virginia
P.O. Box 980118
Richmond, VA 23298

Dr. John H. McGovern
114 E. 72nd Street
New York, NY 10021

Dr. J. William McRoberts
University of Kentucky
Medical School
800 Rose Street
Lexington, KY 40506

Dr. Richard G. Middleton
University of Utah
50 N. Medical Drive
Salt Lake City, UT 84132

Dr. Vincent J. O'Connor
Northwestern Medical School
303 Chicago Avenue
Chicago, IL 60611

Dr. Carl Olsson
The Presbyterian Hospital in
The City of New York
5141 Broadway
New York, NY 10034

Dr. Paul C. Peters
University of Texas
Southwestern Medical School
5323 Harry Hines Boulevard
Dallas, TX 75235

Dr. Victor A. Politano
Jackson Memorial Hospital
1611 NW 12th Avenue
Miami, FL 33136

Dr. Jon M. Reckler
New York Urological Associates
880 Fifth Avenue
New York, NY 10021

Dr. Robert K. Rhamy
Vanderbilt University
Medical Center
1211 W. 22nd Avenue S.
Nashville, TN 37232

Dr. Donald G. Skinner
University of California
at Los Angeles Medical School
10833 Leconte Avenue

Dr. Ralph A. Straffon
Cleveland Clinic
9500 Euclid Avenue
Cleveland, OH 44195

Dr. Nelson Stone
Mt. Sinai Hospital
100th Street
and Madison Avenue
New York, NY 10029

Prostate Cancer Surgeons:

Dr. William R. Fair
Memorial Sloan-Kettering
Cancer Center
1275 York Avenue
New York, NY 10021

Dr. Larry Nathanson
Winthrop University Hospital
259 First Street
Mineola, NY 11501

Dr. Thomas Stamey
Stanford University Hospital
300 Pasteur
Stanford, CA 94305

Dr. David C. Utz
Mayo Clinic
200 SW First Street
Rochester, MN 55905

Dr. R. Keith Waterhouse
Downstate Medical Center
450 Clarkson Avenue
Brooklyn, NY 11203

Dr. Willet F. Whitmore
425 E. 67th Street
New York, NY 10021

Dr. Patrick C. Walsh
Johns Hopkins University
300 Pasteur
Baltimore, MD 21218

Radiation Oncologists:

Dr. Zvi Y. Fuks
Memorial Sloan-Kettering
Cancer Center
1275 York Avenue
New York, NY 10021

Dr. Malcolm A. Bagshaw
Stanford University
Medical Center
300 Pasteur
Stanford, CA 93405

Dr. Luther W. Brady
Hahnemann Medical College
230 N. Broad Street
Philadelphia, PA 19102

Dr. Melvin L. Griem
University of Chicago Hospital
950 E. 59th Street
Chicago, IL 60637

Dr. Samuel Hellman
Harvard Medical School
25 Shattuck Street
Boston, MA 02115

Dr. Henry S. Kaplan
Stanford University
300 Pasteur
Medical Center
Stanford, CA 94305

Dr. Simon Kramer
Thomas Jefferson
Memorial Hospital
111 S. Eleventh Street
Philadelphia, PA 19107

Dr. Fred Lee
Crittenton Hospital
1101 W. University
Rochester, MI 48307

Dr. Seymour Levitt
University of Minnesota
Hospital
420 Delaware Street, SE
Minneapolis, MN 55455

Dr. John G. Maier
Fairfax Hospital
3300 Gallows Road
Falls Church, VA 22046

Dr. William Moss
Oregon Health Sciences Center
3181 SW Sam Jackson Park Rd.
Portland, OR 97201

Dr. Carlos A. Perez
Washington University
School of Medicine
Mallinckrodt Institute of Radiology
510 S. Kings Highway
St. Louis, MO 63110

Dr. Ruheri Perez-Tamayo
Loyola Medical Center
2160 S. First Avenue
Maywood, IL 60153

Dr. William E. Powers
The Harper Grace Hospital
3990 John R.
Detroit, MI 48201

Dr. W.D. Rider
Ontario Cancer Institute
Princess Margaret Hospital
500 Shearbourne Street
Toronto, Ont. Canada M4X 1K9

Dr. Philip Ruben
Strong Memorial Hospital
601 Elmwood Avenue
Rochester, NY 14642

Dr. Jerome Vaeth
St. Mary's Hospital
and Medical Center
2200 Hayes Street
San Francisco, CA 94117

Dr. George Varsos
Rahway Regional Cancer Center
892 Trussler Road
Rahway, NJ 07065

Dr. Michael Zelefsky
Memorial Sloan-Kettering
Cancer Center
1275 York Avenue
New York, NY 10021

Dr. Jeff Forman
Wayne State University
Medical School
540 E. Canfield
Detroit, MI 48201

Dr. Kent Wallner
Memorial Sloan-Kettering
Cancer Center
1275 York Avenue
New York, NY 10021

Medical Oncologists:

Dr. E. Roy Berger
North Shore Hematology/
Oncology Associates, P.C.
267C E. Main Street
Smithtown, NY 11787

Dr. George Bosl
Memorial Sloan-Kettering
Cancer Center
1275 York Avenue
New York, NY 10021

Dr. Lawrence Einhorn
Indiana University
Hospital, Room 1730
550 N. University Blvd
Indianapolis, IN 46202

Dr. Mario Eisenberger
University of Maryland
School of Medicine
655 W. Baltimore Street
Baltimore, MD 21201

Dr. Christopher John Logothetis
M.D. Anderson Cancer Center
1515 Holcombe Boulevard
Houston, TX 77030

Dr. Howard Scher
Memorial Sloan-Kettering
Cancer Center
1275 York Avenue
New York, NY 10021

Dr. Frank Torti   Dr. Alan Yagoda
V.A. Medical Center   Columbia-Presbyterian
3801 Miranda Avenue   Medical Center
Palo Alto, CA 94304   622 W. 168th Street
                                   New York, NY 10032

For the Cost-Conscious

If you cannot afford a doctor to diagnose and treat you for prostate cancer and you are a veteran, there are a number of physicians at Veterans Administration (V.A.) Hospitals around the nation who can diagnose and treat your disease, probably without any cost. Several men in my two prostate cancer sup-port groups were diagnosed, as well as treated, by very competent physicians in V.A. Hospitals and were more than satisfied.

If you are not a veteran and cannot afford a doctor, some community hospitals will enable their doctors to diagnose and treat you, and they will be satisfied with what Medicare reimburses them for the professional service.

The New York Hospital-Cornell Medical Center has opened the Brady Prostate Center for men who cannot afford the cost of going to the doctor to have their prostate examined. Under the direction of Aaron P. Perlmutter, M.D., Ph.D., the Brady Center is a facility that offers men the opportunity for diagnosis and treatment of prostate cancer, as well as providing an access to new prostate medication. The Brady Center offers free prostate evaluation to any man over forty years of age, who meet the criteria for an on-going research srudy, which may include digital rectal examination and PSA blood test. For an appointment, call (212) 746-5359, Monday through Friday, 9 a.m. to 5 p.m.

Members of the American Association of Retired Persons (AARP) can obtain prescription medications through the AARP pharmacy. You may find the cost to be substantially lower than those available at your neighborhood pharmacy.

Alternatively, there are prescription membership organizations that present the possibility of obtaining reduced costs for medications, regardless of whether or not you have prescription reimbursement through medical insurance. A plan such as this could provide benefit to you. The American Preferred Plan (APP) is one such organization. The APP summarizes the advantages for those who have prescription coverage through private insurance, such as Blue Cross/Blue Shield, as follows:

> There is no cost for membership. Members may mail their prescriptions (without any payment), or their physician may call in the prescription directly to the pharmacy (toll free) at (800) 227-1195. Within twenty-four hours, the pharmacy ships the prescription by UPS second-day air at no charge to the patient. If the physician authorizes refills, the medication is shipped with refill slips and postage-paid return envelopes.

> The APP files for reimbursement with the member's insurance company and waits the usual six to eight weeks for payment. No worry or follow up is required by the patient. There is no payment for membership, and no bills are sent to the patient for prescriptions by the pharmacy.

For those who do not have prescription coverage through insurance, the following applies:

> There is no cost for membership. While the patient must pay for his pharmaceuticals, members of PAACT will receive their prescriptions at substantial savings.

> When you call the toll free number (800) 227-1195, you must identify yourself as a member of PAACT, and specify group #395. You will be entered on their computer as such for all further transactions. All of your pharmaceutical requirements (not only flutamide) can be taken care of under this plan, if you wish.

There are other prescription maintenance service organizations that are structured similarly, such as Medical Association of America (MAOA). Contact them at (800) 428-6262 for specific information regarding this plan.

Those who do not have prescription coverage, and meet specific qualifications for low-income patients may be eligible to receive flutamide (Eulexin) through the "Indigent Needs Program" offered by the Schering-Plough Corporation. In order to apply for this program, you must contact your personal physician. Your physician must then contact the local Schering-Plough sales representative who can provide your physician with the necessary application form(s) and instructions.

There are many other drug companies that will make their products available to low-income patients free of charge, provided the patient does not have any other way to pay for the medication. The Pharmaceutical Manufacturers Association has a publication available (to physicians only) that currently lists fifty-nine prescription drug Indigent Needs Programs. The medications available are not restricted to those used in prostate cancer therapy.

Qualification procedures vary from one pharmaceutical company to another. Physicians can obtain up-to-date information about which drugs are available, as well as application procedures for patients, by requesting the free publications, "Directory of Prescription Drug Indigent Programs" from the Pharmaceutical Manufacturers Association, 1100 Fifteenth Street NW, Washington DC 20005. Your doctor can also obtain information by calling (800) PMA-INFO.

Questions to Ask Your Physician

After you have become knowledgeable about the diagnosis and treatment of prostate cancer, establish a list of questions to determine if the doctor is abreast of new trends, changes, and developments in prostate cancer treatment. Use a list of questions similar to the following to interview and select your doctor:

a. What are your thoughts in recommending combination hormonal therapy as an initial treatment for most stages of prostate cancer?

b. How would you determine watchful waiting patients?

c. Would you recommend cryosurgery for one of your patients when radiation failed? Why?

d. Would you recommend estrogen over flutamide? Why?

The appropriate responses to these questions are as follows:

a. Yes, I am in favor of using combination hormonal therapy as a preliminary treatment for prostate cancer when it is desirable to downstage the tumor to make it more manageable for treatment.

b. I would develop a list of criteria that would include age, acceptable PSA level, Gleason score, and proper stage, and require a diploid DNA study.

c. Yes, and if that failed, I would treat him again with cryosurgery and/or place him on combination hormonal therapy.

d. Absolutely not. There are some terrible side effects of estrogen; luprolide and flutamide have less threatening side effects.

Request your family doctor to recommend a doctor to you, and when he or she does, follow up with this statement: "Would you send your father to this doctor? Why?" If you are satisfied with your doctor's response, proceed. You could also ask your doctor to identify three or four other doctors of the same discipline, interview each one, and make a selection. You could identify some of the prominent men or women in the country who have been exposed to a large number of doctors through visitations at hospitals and attendance at professional seminars and conferences to recommend doctors to you. To this end, I contacted Ney of PAACT to recommend an oncologist to me. He made his recommendation, I made an appointment to meet with the doctor he recommended, and I was satisfied.

Figure 5.1
Checklist for Selecting Your Doctor

Humanity	Yes	No
1. Does your doctor use the sense of touch when he or she greets you?	_____	_____
2. When he or she completes discussing a "sensitive issue" with you, does he or she bring or put an arm around your shoulder?	_____	_____
3. Does your doctor explain to you a procedure before and during the process?	_____	_____
4. Does your doctor apologize for hurting you or making you uncomfortable?	_____	_____
5. Does your doctor use simple words and explain medical terms when conversing with you?	_____	_____
6. Is your doctor considerate of the whole you, that is, does he or she view you as a human being rather than a "prostate gland" to be treated?	_____	_____
7. Does your doctor consider you a partner and respect your right to make diagnostic and treatment dicisions contrary to his or hers?	_____	_____
8. Does your doctor mind when you question his or her advice or recommendations?	_____	_____

If your assessment reveals a high number of "No" answers in any category, I strongly suggest you get another doctor.

Based on some of my research and reading, I have arrived at the checklist illustrated in Figure 5.1 to offer you a more comprehensive way to select your doctor. The checklist is only a suggestion and you need not answer all of the questions. Select those you feel are important. Obviously, some questions are more important than others, so read through the entire list first.

Figure 5.1 (Continued)
Checklist for Selecting Your Doctor

Qualifications	Yes	No
1. Is your doctor board certified?	_____	_____
2. Is your doctor willing to give you the names of patients he or she has operated on or performed some sort of professional service for as referrals?	_____	_____
3. Has your doctor ever participated in any clinical trials?	_____	_____
4. Does your doctor's office display his or her degrees and advanced certificates?	_____	_____
5. Is your doctor affiliated with one of the top hospitals in the community? (Top hospitals are decided by being among the top three to five.)	_____	_____
6. Has your doctor published any professional articles?	_____	_____
7. Is your doctor aware of some of the recent trends and developments in his or her field?	_____	_____
8. Are your satisfied with how your doctor communicates with you?	_____	_____
9. Does your doctor have a good reputaion among his or her peers?	_____	_____
10. Have you checked the Directory of Medical Specialists to review the backround of your doctor?	_____	_____

COMMUNICATING WITH YOUR DOCTOR

At the Oncology Division of the Albany Medical College in New York, a study was performed in which researchers followed oncologists on their morning tours and observed and denoted everything the doctors said to their patients. Subsequent to the study, the researchers followed up with interviews with the patients to determine what the doctors did to enable them to feel that their needs were being met. The study concluded that the one thing the patients wanted more than anything else was information. This portion of the chapter will describe what value you can get from talking to your doctor, how to enhance the communication process, why you may fail to communicate to your doctor, and what you can do if you find it difficult to do so.

Most patients who go to their doctors for either diagnosis or treatment tend to be timid and reluctant to question them. They tend to acquiesce to their doctor's "professional training," knowledge, and experience. Decisions are usually made in a dictatorial mode; that is, the physician makes most of the medical decisions for the patient. The patient sits as a passive individual leaving the fate of his or her life in the hands of the competent or incompetent doctor. I maintain that it should not to be like that. The relationship between the patient and physician should be similar to a partnership in which each opinion and judgement is respected, and decisions are made in a democratic manner. With these thoughts, I used the following principles to govern any behavior with my doctor.

- When visiting my doctor for diagnosis or treatment, my approach was that he or she is the professional provider and I am the patient; therefore, I am the boss—he or she is not my boss.

- I was not afraid to ask my doctors questions, even though the questions may have seemed stupid.

- I was guided by my Prostate Cancer Report Card when asking my doctor questions.

- I asked my doctor to explain any procedure performed on me. For example, if he took my blood pressure, I wanted to know the reading. If he listened to my heart, I would inquire about my heart rate. If he took my blood, I asked him why. If he took a test for my PSA level, I asked him to report the level to me (usually after several days).

- I do not hesitate to show off my knowledge about my prostate condition. My doctors respect me for this behavior and I respect myself.

What Value Will You Get From Talking to Your Doctor?

J.B. was told by his doctor that his blood test revealed he has prostate cancer. His doctor told him that it was detected early, so if he got an operation immediately, his life would be saved. J.B. was terrified and consented to the surgery. Several months after the operation, he went to a support group and there he recognized that he had acted on the doctor's recommendation in haste. You see, J.B. was 70 years old and had suffered from a heart attack several months earlier. J.B. could have spared himself an operation, one that could have cost him his life, if he had talked to his doctor and asked him several questions, or if he had gotten a second, and even a third opinion.

Most doctors would not have operated on J.B. because of his heart condition and his age. What did J.B. do wrong? He let his emotions get the best of him without exploring his condition and the various options for treatment. He let one doctor, a urologist who makes his living by operating on people, decide on a treatment for his prostate disease. If J.B. had waited and thoroughly researched and read the various literature available to him; contacted various support groups, such as US TOO and PAACT, and talked to other prostate cancer sufferers; and became familiar with information about prostate cancer, I am certain he would not have allowed the doctor to operate on him. With knowledge, his timidity would have been replaced by confidence. Such confidence would have propelled him to challenge his doctor, ask him several questions, and subsequently, to get another opinion. Remember, I got three opinions from different urologists before I finally decided on a treatment protocol. Notice, I said *I* decided on a treatment protocol. Once you gain information about your condition and prostate cancer, you are in an improved position to make appropriate choices. You are less inclined to let one doctor decide your fate. No one has a greater stake in your fate than you; not your doctor, mother, nor anyone. You are the captain of your ship.

Although we have touched on the options available to J.B., let us review all of them. I have already mentioned watchful waiting; however, he could have also opted for either combination hormonal therapy or radiation treatment. He might have learned that an operation is not advisable because of his heart condition. He could have requested a DNA study to determine the type of prostate cancer cells he had to verify a watchful waiting decision.

As you can glean from the above information, J.B. would have been more in control of his fate with the acquisition of knowledge and information. Instead, he put his entire life in the hands of a doctor who should have known that a person who has had a heart attack a few months previously is not a good candidate for a radical prostatectomy.

You might say, suppose my doctor refuses to give me information, how will I know what to do? Politely tell him or her that you need information in order to make a decision and that you must get that information from at least two different doctors. State that you have listened to his or her recommendations and reasons for these, and now must listen to another doctor's opinions.

What You Can Do to Enhance the Communication Process With Your Doctor

When going to your doctor to either find out your condition or discuss other particulars pertaining to prostate cancer, write down a list of appropriate questions. The following is such a list. When your doctor recommends a specific choice of treatment, you should ask:

- What is my last PSA level, Gleason score, stage, DNA study results, and the results of other studies?

- Do I need additional tests? If yes, why?

- Why do you recommend this treatment as opposed to other treatments?

- What will happen if I choose not to take your recommended treatment?

- Will your choice of treatment cure my condition, shrink my prostate gland, or palliate my disease?

- Why do you recommend this treatment?

- What other traditional and nontraditional treatments are available and why do you not favor them?

- What is the cost? Is it approved by my insurance company?

- What are the possible side effects of treatment?

- Do you mind if I get a second opinion?

Once you have considered the above questions and added your own, give a copy to your wife and family members and request that they add questions to the list.

Why You May Find It Difficult to Talk to Your Doctor

A support group on prostate cancer at the Memorial Sloan-Kettering Cancer Center brainstormed the following reasons used by patients who found it difficult to communicate to their doctors. I am presenting them to give you food for thought to open up your communication processes.

The number-one reason was the belief that doctors are too busy to allocate time for their patients to communicate to them. Even if this may not be true, many of the group members felt it is true; therefore, it is a problem that both patients and doctors must deal with.

Fear was a trait that received a great deal of attention. Members felt that because they lacked information, they did not know what to ask. Rather than seem like a "dummy," they settled for acquiescing to their doctor's advisement.

Some said that they were too shocked to ask questions. Concern for their personal welfare plus the lack of information immobilized them.

Doctors' social power and social level were two subjects that were discussed. It appears that some of the patients with prostate cancer felt that they do not know how to relate to the social power that doctors carry with them. Neither are some doctors able to relate to their patients. I believe this problem seems to be inherent with those patients who may not be college graduates and are threatened by the doctor's information base. There may be something to this. As a result of my education and the knowledge I have accumulated in response to my personal needs and this book, I did not feel in the least threatened by "doctors' social power or social level."

Some of the participants in the group felt that they found it difficult to relate to the doctors because of the special language they use, including terms like PSA level, Gleason, stage, prostatectomy, carcinoma, and metastasize.

Lack of questions was also discussed. Members felt because they had a lack of information pertaining to their condition, as well as to prostate cancer, they could not ask intelligent questions.

Doctor's adult or parent ego versus the patient's child ego was also a factor in why patients found it difficult to talk to their doctors. Some doctors talked down to them. However, some members felt that this was changing to some extent.

Some members of the support group felt that it was routine for some doctors to make it difficult for patients to relate to them. This was usually a result of those doctors coming from larger hospitals where impersonality was a standard mode, particularly those who saw thousands of patients each year.

Some members felt that just the mere fact that doctors know more than the patient made the patient feel subservient to the doctor and made it difficult to relate to them based on their limited knowledge base.

What You Can Do If You Find It Difficult to Communicate to Your Doctor

First and foremost, if you find it difficult to communicate to your doctor, educate yourself by the various means discussed in this chapter and throughout this book. Prior to making an appointment with your doctor to discuss your case, jot down your questions and let one of your colleagues review your list to determine if you have omitted any. The questions in this chapter are an excellent source from which to begin. If you have joined a support group, circulate the list among the members for discussion and add to the list.

Prepare an agenda as a guide to conduct your discussion with your doctor. Consider some of the questions in this chapter as agenda items. Take along a tape recorder to record your discussion with your doctor. Jot down your doctor's answers if he or she feels uncomfortable with the tape recorder. Bring someone with you, either your wife, another relative, or an acquaintance. This person may be able to ask questions that you have not thought of. When my doctor was about to report all the results of my tests and recommend a treatment, I brought along my wife and my sister. Furthermore, I maintained a copy of all my records in my personal files. I frequently serve as a prostate cancer confidante by appearing with prostate cancer patients at their physician's office and asking pertinent questions on their behalf; explaining tests and procedures; and providing them with information so they can decide on a treatment of choice. If you can get someone to act as your prostate cancer confidante, it can relieve you of a great deal of anxiety.

Questions You Should Ask Your Doctor Regarding Radical Prostatectomy

If your doctor recommends radical prostatectomy, you should ask:

- What surgical approach (perineal or retropubic) will you use? Why?

- Do you have any experience in the nerve-sparing surgery? How many patients have you treated with this surgery technique? What percentage of your patients remains potent after the operation?
- Can you give me the names and telephone numbers of six patients for me to interview on whom you have operated? (Some physicians will and others will not.)
- What is my risk if I do not have surgery?
- Will you personally perform the operation?
- What are the potential side effects and what is the probability that I will have them?
- Will I receive any other treatments prior to and/or after surgery?
- Will I become incontinent? For about how long? Will I have to wear an adult diaper?
- How will you accommodate any pain I might have?
- What adjustments will I have to make in my daily activities after surgery? For how long following surgery?
- How long will it be before I can perform sexually?
- How long will it be before I am fully cured of the disease?
- What is the probability that my disease will not recur?
- How long will I be in the hospital? Which hospital?

Questions You Should Ask Your Doctors Regarding External Beam Radiation or Seed Implantation

If your doctor recommends external beam radiation or seed implantation therapy, you should ask:

- Why are you recommending external beam radiation therapy as opposed to radical prostatectomy or seed implantation?
- How many treatments will I need and how long will each treatment be?

- What are the side effects? Which ones will I most likely get?
- How is quality control monitored to ensure that the radiation beam is actually concentrated on the appropriate sites?
- Will I receive any other treatment prior to, during, and/or after radiation treatment?
- Will I be able to schedule the treatment to accommodate my daily activities?
- What are the consequences if I miss a treatment?
- Are there any risks? What are these?
- How many rads (unit measure of radiation) will I get? How did you decide how many I will receive?
- Can I have radical prostatectomy if radiation fails to cure my disease?
- Can I have the names and telephone numbers of six of your patients who have had radiation therapy?
- What percentage of your patients have had a recurrence of the disease after treatment?

Questions You Should Ask Your Doctors Regarding Specific Treatments

In an effort to assist you in asking your doctors pointed questions pertaining to your choice of treatment, I have identified the following for your consideration. Others may also be included. If your doctor recommends combination hormonal therapy or chemotherapy, you should ask:

- What specific hormones or drugs will you use?
- How much of the hormone will I be administered per day?
- How often will I need to take the medication?
- What will happen if I miss taking the hormone or drug?
- What are the side effects?

- Do I need to be put on a special diet?
- What other drugs should I avoid when taking the hormone or drug?
- What are the consequences if I do not take hormonal therapy or chemotherapy?
- Will my sex life be affected by the hormone or drug?
- What has been the success rate of the hormone or drug?
- Will you give me the names and telephone numbers of patients who were treated with either hormones or drugs?

Study the Patient's Bill of Rights

The American Hospital Association has prepared a Patient's Bill of Rights with the expectation that observance of these rights will help provide improved care and satisfaction for the patient by the physician and hospital. It maintains that a personal relationship between the doctor and the patient is essential for providing proper medical care. There are twelve provisions of these rights as discussed below:

1. This provision maintains that proper and respectful medical care is a fundamental right of every patient.
2. Freedom of information is the key provision here. If it is not advisable to give the information directly to the patient, then the information should be given to someone else in his or her behalf. (Because most patients do not know their rights, they are not aware that they have a right to review the medical chart that is maintained on all patients. The provision also gives you the right to ask for a copy of all your medical records from your doctor.)
3. This provision contains the clause "informed consent," but it is not practiced by many doctors. Informed consent basically means that the doctor has no rights to treat you unless you have been "properly" informed.
4. All patients have the right not to accept the recommendation of the doctor, but the doctor has a right to inform the

patient of the consequences of not accepting his or her recommendation.

5. This provision protects the privacy rights of the patient. The release of patient records without his or her consent is forbidden.

6. Provision six is similar to the previous provision, but goes further and specifies "all communications."

7. This provision maintains that the hospital must be prompt in response to a patient's request for services. Also, the hospital cannot transfer the patient without giving him reasons why the transfer must be made.

8. In this provision, the patient has the right to get information pertaining to the relationship of the hospital with other institutions if related to his medical case, as well as information pertaining to personal relationships.

9. In this provision, no hospital can use the patient in experimentation without his or her consent.

10. This provision ensures that the patient has a right for continuous care, either in the hospital or at home. In essence, the patient's physician or a delegate must be on call in the event of a need.

11. This provision ensures that the patient has a right to receive an adequate explanation pertaining to medical charges.

12. Lastly, the patient has the right to review the Code of Conduct for the patient, that is, what is expected of the patient.

HOW YOU CAN GET INFORMATION
ON PROSTATE CANCER

There are a multitude of techniques to gain information on prostate cancer. Most of these will be discussed in this chapter. Knowledge is power. When you use each of these techniques, you are basically arming yourself to communicate to your doctor, to put yourself on the same level as your doctor, and to protect your life from unscrupulous doctors. True, you will find that the more information you acquire, the more confused you will become. However, it is better to have too much information than to have too little to make a decision.

Support groups, such as US TOO, PAACT, and local support groups that are affiliated with large hospitals are good sources to meet other victims of prostate cancer, as well as to listen to them for information and to learn of their choices of treatment. An organization like PAACT that is involved in reporting and conducting research on prostate cancer is an invaluable support group for patients with prostate cancer, as I reported in Chapter Four.

Newsletters about prostate cancer are an excellent source to acquire information. Two of the popular ones are *Cancer Communication*, published by PAACT, and the *US TOO Newsletter*, published by US TOO. Some medical schools and hospitals also publish newsletters related to prostate cancer. Books are also excellent resources to read about the diagnosis and treatment for prostate cancer. The bibliography in the back of books is a good source for obtaining additional materials on the subject. Recently I purchased a textbook on prostate cancer entitled *Cancer of the Prostate*. Although I found the book extremely informative, I did have to use a dictionary at times and the glossary of terms to fully understand the contents.

Conferences are a good source for gaining current information on prostate cancer. However, not many prostate cancer patients attend such meetings. I think this is because they feel that the information is too technical for them. I know PAACT periodically sponsors symposiums. Some prostate cancer patients have been known to attend conferences sponsored by professional associations of physicians.

The electronic mailboxes of PAACT and of several hospitals in the nation are an invaluable source for gaining information on various topics related to prostate cancer. Once when I was reading a publication of PAACT, I did not quite understand an article about the DNA ploidy analysis study, so I went to my telephone and dialed the appropriate number and listened to a presentation of DNA ploidy analysis. By establishing a telephone network with other patients with prostate cancer, you can gain a great deal of insight into the disease. To establish your network, acquire a membership with US TOO and/or PAACT and ask them to share the membership list with you. If they do not have a policy of sharing their membership list, ask them to publish an article relating to your desire to establish a telephone network on prostate cancer.

PROTECTING YOURSELF AGAINST
MEDICAL MISTAKES

In 1991, the *New England Journal of Medicine* reported that in 1984, standard operating procedure harmed nearly 100,000 and killed more than 13,000 people in New York state alone. Think about what the procedure could cause people in all the 50 states. If we make a projection on a national scale, this means that medical mistakes and malpractice might have caused harm to 1.4 million Americans, killing about 186 thousand in just one year.

This is why I have devoted Chapter Nine to a holistic approach for treating your prostate cancer condition once your medical treatment has been completed. Things are changing so drastically in various allied fields that it is important for you to stay abreast of traditional and nontraditional treatments, enhanced medical technology and procedures, and of various other areas such as herbal medicine, acupuncture, and other tools of healing.

The following are suggestions to protect yourself from medical mistakes:

1. Do not passively accept any diagnosis or treatment without fortifying yourself with knowledge and knowing your alternatives.

2. Treat your physician the same way you treat any other professional whom you pay for a service.

3. If your physician does not have sufficient time for you to have a discussion about your diagnosis and treatment, get another doctor.

4. Although you should consider recommendations by your physician, your destiny is in your hands. You should decide what is best for you and your family.

5. Once you have armed yourself with information, join a prostate cancer support group to listen to your colleagues, interact with numerous physicians, and consider using your instincts to make a treatment decision.

6. Get three, four, or even five professional opinions on treatment until you are satisfied.

7. Collect sources on the best doctors in the nation and start from these to select your doctors.

8. Remain abreast of the latest research on prostate cancer.

If you have been diagnosed with prostate cancer, one of the most important tasks will be to make a decision as to the doctor(s) who will treat you. You must do this deliberately. Do not just settle for your doctor's choice. Investigate your doctor regarding his choice and then do some research and ask others. Once you have selected several doctors, use the checklist to rank each doctor. When you have made a choice of treatment, discuss it with your doctor and try to reach a consensus. Use the remaining names in the event you need a second or third opinion. When you go to your doctor to hear what he or she has to say about your prostate condition, go around with specific questions to ask him or her. If your doctor recommends a specific treatment, you should also be prepared to ask him or her relevant questions to help you make up your mind.

Regardless of the approach you use in selecting a physician, you should thoroughly check his or her credentials. Prepare a list of questions with which to interview your doctor. Observe the office staff to determine if they are "on top of things." I remember an incident when the office staff failed to deliver important papers to another doctor, causing a significant loss of time for treatment.

As mentioned previously, if you cannot find a doctor to diagnose and treat your prostate cancer, there are a number of organizations and hospitals that will do so for men who are in need.

Throughout this book, I have stated when I believe a medical mistake has been made in regard to either my diagnosis and/or treatment. Profit from my experience and use the substance of this book to guard against medical mistakes.

CHAPTER SIX

Thank God For Flutamide

Eight years ago, Lloyd Ney walked into his doctor's office and was told he had an advanced stage of prostate cancer and had only three to six months to live. Five years ago, M.L. was shocked when he was informed by his doctor that he had only four months to live. This year, J.B. was told he had cancer and should go straight to his lawyer to make out his will. Since then, thousands of patients who were suffering from an advanced stage of prostate cancer are alive thanks to Ney, the aforementioned executive director of PAACT, and a group of physicians who convinced the FDA to approve a drug called flutamide (Eulexin is the brand name) which, when used in combination with luprolide, has either saved or lengthened the lives of hundreds of thousands of patients with prostate cancer.

Cancer cells thrive on testosterone. To produce testosterone, the body needs to produce a naturally occurring substance called luteinizing hormone-releasing hormone or LHRH. Synthetic substances similar to LHRH are luprolide and zoladex. Once per month, 7.5 milligrams of luprolide or 3.6 milligrams of zoladex is injected into either the buttocks or the abdominal muscle to halt the production of testosterone from the testes.

Flutamide is an antiandrogen substance that can counteract the biological effects of the hormones in cells located in the body that depend in some manner on androgens. Flutamide is of the non-steroidal type. The recommended dose is 250 mg every eight hours.

Flutamide works at the site of hormonally-dependent pros-tate cancer cells by preventing the adrenal androgens from being used as a source for nourishing them. Therefore, cancer cells are attacked at two levels: at the testes, using luprolide; and in the adrenal glands, using flutamide. The usual side ef-fects are nausea, vomiting, diarrhea, and rarely, altered liver functions. When flutamide is used in combination hormonal therapy, the side effects are bloating, diarrhea, and hot flashes. In my case, I also got brown spots on the bald part of my head and frequent incidents of flatulence.

Is flutamide, when used in combination with luprolide (called combination hormonal therapy), a miracle drug? I do not know. In fact, most doctors do not believe it is a cure for prostate cancer. I can say, however, that it has been used as a diagnostic agent; as a preliminary treatment for most stages of prostate cancer; as an early treatment for prostate cancer; as an effective agent for downstaging and debulking prostate can-cer; as a viable option for surgical castration; as an effective agent to improve survival time and prolong life; and as an effective agent even after relapse. Each one of these benefits will be discussed below.

LUPROLIDE AND FLUTAMIDE
AS A DIAGNOSTIC AGENT

When I was diagnosed with prostate cancer, I was Stage B/C after a biopsy. To determine if the disease had spread, my doc-tor ordered a CT scan and a bone scan. The results of these two tests revealed that there were some spots on the films of both tests. The radiation oncologist's report was inconclusive: It said the spots could have been the result of carcinoma or Paget's disease. So, my doctor ordered a skeletal survey and bone biopsy.

The skeletal survey proved very little. The bone biopsy was negative. My doctor then requested that I go to Memorial Sloan-Kettering Cancer Center and meet with Harry Herr, M.D., whom we both agreed on. Dr. Herr suggested that I be put on combination hormonal therapy for a period of three months. After that, a new CT scan would be performed. If these spots were not visible on the film of the new CT scan, then it would be evident that the combination hormonal therapy had worked, suggesting carcinoma.

On the other hand, if the spots remained visible on the film of the new CT scan, then it would be evident that the disease had not spread throughout my body. Fortunately for me, the spots remained on the film, suggesting they were from Paget's disease. However, my oncologist and one of his associates were not convinced and suggested that I get an MRI, which I did. The report from the radiation oncologist indicated Paget's disease.

These tests proved that combination hormonal therapy can be effectively used to diagnose if prostate cancer has spread into the bones of a patient. Spots on the film of a CT scan or bone scan can also be attributed to Paget's disease, arthritis, or some other bone disease. I see no reason why this technique cannot be used on patients when there is a suspicion that the disease has spread to human organs.

LUPROLIDE AND FLUTAMIDE AS A PRELIMINARY TREATMENT FOR MOST STAGES OF PROSTATE CANCER

Stage A

In Stage A1, there is pathological evidence of prostate cancer, and there are no more than three well-differentiated tumors. Because your disease is nonbulky, you may not need combination hormonal therapy. In addition, this may be the stage in which you may be classified as a "watchful waiting" candidate.

In Stage A2, there is also pathological evidence of prostate cancer.

There are either more than three well-differentiated tumors or any growth of higher-grade tumors. Your physician may decide to shrink an enlarged prostate using combination hormonal therapy to make it more manageable for treatment and/or to capitalize on other benefits of this therapy as cited in Stage B.

Stage B

In Stage B, prostate cancer is clinically confirmed by a biopsy and is confined to the prostate on digital rectal examination.

During this stage of prostate cancer when the tumor is bulky, combination hormonal therapy is used to debulk the prostate gland to make it more manageable for treatment. This is true if the treatment is radical prostatectomy, external beam radiation, or most other treatments. Combination hormonal therapy reduces morbidity and blood loss, makes dissection easier, facilitates complete removal of the gland and other cancerous tissues and organs, and minimizes side effects In a randomized trial, for patients utilizing three months of combination hormonal therapy prior to radical prostatectomy, marginal disease was reduced from 38.5 percent to only 13 percent.

In addition, when the final stage of the disease was determined through an examination of the biopsied specimen and compared to the one estimated previously, it was discovered that a more advanced stage (upstaging of the disease) was found in 53.8 percent of the control patients. Therefore, 23.4 percent of the patients receiving combination hormonal therapy achieved a more favorable stage than that determined initially (downstaging), thus showing a marked advantage of 77.2 percent in favor of the patients receiving combination hormonal therapy.

As reported previously, there is one exception to this claim that combination hormonal therapy should precede all stages of treatment for prostate cancer. My radiation oncologist indicates that combination hormonal therapy has been very instrumental in debulking large prostate glands; however, he maintains that it has little value in treating early stage non-bulky tumors.

Combination hormonal therapy is proving effective with Stage B and C patients. Pilepich Miljenko, M.D. of Ann Arbor, Michigan conducted a study whereby 30 patients staged B or C were administered zoladex (a substitute for luprolide) and flutamide two months prior to radiation treatment. With a minimum follow up of two years, the primary lesions were cleared of the disease in 25 of 30 patients.

Stage C

In Stage C, the cancer has spread beyond the prostate gland to the tissue immediately around it.

In the same study, 67 untreated Stage C patients received combination hormonal therapy. Treatment continued for an average of 23.5 months. At two years, only 5 patients showed treatment failure with a probability of continuous response of 91.8 percent. Three patients died from prostate cancer and three died of other causes for a probable survival rate of 93.5 percent at 2 years. When comparing results with treatment with a single hormone, castration, or radiation, the rate of treatment failure at 2 years is 3.5-fold lower after combination hormonal therapy (8.2 percent) than monotherapy, or a single treatment (28.4 percent). The probability of death at 2 years following the beginning of combination hormonal therapy is 6.5 percent, while it is an average of 22.2 percent (3.4 times higher) in studies using monotherapy.

PAACT maintains that combination hormonal therapy has shown to be effective in treating patients whose prostate cancer has spread to the bones and that even better results can be obtained when it is used earlier, namely at Stage C of the disease, before clinical evidence that the disease has spread to the bones.

Stage D

In Stage D, the cancer has spread to the lymph nodes, bones, and other organs.

In a Canadian study (Beland, et.al.), the percentage of Stage D patients who did not respond to castration was 39 percent. This percentage decreased to 16 percent in Stage D patients who received luprolide in addition to surgical orchiectomy. The percentage of patients not responding was further decreased to 9 percent in those receiving combination hormonal therapy, representing a 23.4 percent advantage over castration alone.

In 1985, a trial was supported by the National Cancer Institute to test the effectiveness of combination hormonal therapy. The study involved 603 untreated Stage D2 patients. Of the 603 patients, 303 were randomly assigned to receive combination hormonal therapy and 300 were assigned to receive luprolide plus a placebo. The group receiving combination hormonal therapy was free of progression of the disease by 16.5 months versus 13.9 months, and overall survival was 35.6 months versus 28.3 months. However, patients with minimal disease, i.e., in the skeleton, pelvis, and soft tissues, experienced a more significant benefit. Among the 82 patients who had good performance status with minimal disease, the median time before progression of the disease was 19.1 months and the median survival time was 39.6 months for the group treated with monotherapy (perhaps luprolide). The group of patients receiving combination hormonal therapy enjoyed a median time before progression of the disease of 58.3 months and median survival time of 61 months.

It is not surprising that PAACT maintains that "combination hormonal therapy is the first treatment shown to prolong life in prostate cancer."

LUPROLIDE AND FLUTAMIDE AS AN EFFECTIVE AGENT IN EARLY TREATMENT FOR PROSTATE CANCER

In a study by Dr. Labrie, et al., entitled "Major Advantages of Early Administration of Endocrine Combination Therapy in Advanced Prostate Cancer," 286 men with advanced prostate cancer were evaluated according to the number of lesions each had. Bone lesions were present for 261 men, while the remaining ones had prostate cancer in their soft tissue. The 261 patients were organized into three groups: 1) those with 1 to 5 lesions; 2) those with 6 to 20 lesions; and 3) those with 11 to 40 lesions. All patients received combination hormonal therapy, with the exception of 11 who were orchiectomized and received flutamide. In April 1992, 260 patients were eligible for assessment. Of these patients, 80 had a complete response to the combination hormonal therapy, and 75 and 87 patients showed partial and stable responses, respectively. Only 17 patients showed no response. Other causes were responsible for the deaths of 123 patients, thus leaving 111 patients alive. When survival time is analyzed in terms of the severity of the disease at the beginning of the treatment, it is apparent that patients with minimal disease according to clinical symptoms, as well as those who have a small number of bone lesions, had a much better chance for long-term survival.

The median survival time calculated for the group of patients who had minimal symptoms was 5.47 years as compared to 2.71 for those with moderate symptoms or 2.1 years for those who displayed severe symptoms. The significance of this study is that the median survival time was not reduced at 8 years in the group of patients who had 1 to 5 bone lesions, while it was reduced to 3.56 years when the bone lesions increased to 6 to 10 in number. This represents a difference in overall survival time of more than 4.4 years. For patients having 10 to 40 bone lesions, the calculated median survival time was 2.36 years.

This study clearly demonstrates a dramatic difference in life expectancy when combination hormonal therapy is administered early in prostate cancer patients who have 1 to 5 bone metastases, as compared to those who have more than 5 bone lesions. In fact, for the group of patients with one to five bone lesions, the calculated survival time is at least 4.4 years longer than for those patients with 6 to 10 bone lesions. It should be clear from this study that the addition of a small number of bone lesions has a major impact on patient survival time. When the number of bone lesions goes beyond 5, combination hormonal therapy has less of an impact on the duration of survival, thus demonstrating that delaying treatment of advanced prostate cancer is not the prudent thing to do.

Dr. Crawford, et.al., have reported that patients who have minimal disease displayed a much better response to combination hormonal therapy. In fact, a recent analysis by the Intergroup National Cancer Institute revealed an advantage of 19.5 months in survival time for patients with minimal disease who received combination hormonal therapy versus luprolide and a placebo. The median survival time of the whole group of patients was improved. It has also been reported that patients with one or two lesions have a survival time that is much longer than those with more than two lesions.

LUPROLIDE AND FLUTAMIDE AS AN AGENT FOR DOWNSTAGING AND DEBULKING PROSTATE CANCER

Downstaging is the process of reducing the tumor volume in prostate cancer patients sufficiently to affect a decrease in the stage classification of the disease. Debulking the prostate is the process of reducing the volume of the disease in its present location. As soon as the patient begins the combination hormonal therapy, his disease is being treated. As a result, his tumor growth is halted and begins to shrink and his PSA level begins to decrease. When a prostate cancer patient has been on combination hormonal therapy for a period of three months, his prostate volume may decrease by approximately 50 percent and his tumor volume may be reduced as much as 80 percent. In fact, in some instances, downstaging has been so effective that in some patients no signs of tumor involvement have been found when the gland is removed by surgery.

During the fourth International Symposium on Transrectal Ultrasound in the Diagnosis and Management of Prostate Cancer, 1989, Dr. Monfete and colleagues indicated that there was an absence of any signs of residual cancer in 24 percent of patients treated with 3 months of preoperative combination hormonal therapy. In addition, 28 percent of the patients had detectable improvement in the characteristics of the tissue, while no change was observed in 40 percent of the patients. Although there was a decreased level of differentiation in 8 percent of the patients, there were no signs of local or advanced progression of the cancer.

Flutamide in combination with luprolide has also been found to be effective in downstaging localized prostate cancer. Dr. Labrie, the developer of combination hormonal therapy, has conducted research on the value of combination hormonal therapy in early stage patients by utilizing radical prostatectomy as a benchmark for evaluation purposes. Many doctors are still reluctant to treat early stage patients with prostate cancer. More importantly, 40 to 50 percent of the patients who are diagnosed with early stage cancer; that is, their cancer has been confined to the gland, have been found to be understaged when the tumor was examined after surgery. As a result, these patients are at risk in terms of recurrence of the cancer.

A randomized trial utilizing three months of combination hormonal therapy prior to radical prostatectomy reduced the cancer positive margin from 38.5 percent to 13.0 percent. The trial diminished any marginal cancer lying outside of the gland. This was determined from an examination of the tumor that was compared with estimated clinical original staging. A more advanced stage of the disease (upstaging) was found in 53 percent of the control patients as compared to 23.4 percent of those who received (downstaging) combination hormonal therapy. As a result, those who received the combination hormonal therapy showed a significant advantage of 77.2 percent in the form of combination hormonal therapy.

LUPROLIDE AND FLUTAMIDE AS A VIABLE OPTION TO SURGICAL CASTRATION

In 1941, researchers (Huggins, et al., *Journal of Urology*, 1940-43: 705-714) found that prostate cancer is dependent on male hormones, androgens, for growth and stimulation. As discussed previously, in men, the primary source of hormones is testosterone, which is produced by the testicles. As a result, testosterone can be halted by removing the testes through surgery, a procedure called orchiectomy, as explained in Chapter Two. However, it should be remembered that the removal of testes does not entirely halt the production of testosterone, because the adrenal glands also produce this hormone.

It appears that 60 to 80 percent of surgically castrated patients showed only a temporary improvement, while 20 to 40 percent of the patients did not experience any improvement in their disease. In addition, those who did experience some improvement after treatment usually showed recurrence of the cancer between 6 to 24 months later. More importantly, when the cancer did recur, the prognosis was extremely gloomy: 50 percent of the patients died within 6 months. As a result, monotherapy; that is, surgical removal of the testes or use of luprolide alone, is insufficient to totally halt the production of testosterone, because these treatments only suppress the male hormones produced by the testes. But, what about the male hormones that are produced by the adrenal glands? Obviously, something must be done to prevent this gland from releasing male hormones. Not only is surgery inadequate, but it is not the only means with which to remove testosterone from the body. Combination hormonal therapy can also remove testosterone and it can do a better job.

Two randomized studies have shown the advantages of using flutamide in combination with luprolide over surgical castration. However, doctors still continue the practice of performing unnecessary surgery on patients with advanced prostate cancer. In a Canadian study (Dr. Beland, et al.), the percentage of patients who did not respond to castration was 39 percent; when a group of patients received flutamide in addition to surgical orchiectomy, the percentage of patients who did not respond to medical and surgical castration was 16 percent. However, when luprolide and flutamide were used in combination, only 9 percent of the patients did not respond to medical castration, representing a 23.4 percent advantage over surgical castration alone. In another study by Dr. Namer in France, 24 percent of advanced stage prostate cancer patients did not respond to surgical castration alone, while only 9 percent of the patients did not respond where flutamide was combined with surgical castration.

LUPROLIDE AND FLUTAMIDE AS AN EFFECTIVE AGENT EVEN AFTER RELAPSE

The median time of survival of 50 percent of the patients who relapse after they begin treatment with monotherapy is expected to be 4 to 9 months. In one study by Dr. Labrie of 266 patients in this category who were administered combination hormonal therapy after relapse, the median time of survival was 13.4 months or 5.3 months longer than the results achieved in a similar group of patients using other treatments. In another study of 126 patients who failed combination hormonal therapy after failing monotherapy, the median survival time was 11 months as compared to 16.3 months for relapsing patients who received combination hormonal therapy as a first treatment.

LUPROLIDE AND FLUTAMIDE AS AN AGENT TO IMPROVE SURVIVAL TIME AND PROLONG LIFE

In 1982, 191 previously untreated patients with advanced stage prostate cancer took part in a multicenter study. The patients received combination hormonal therapy as a first treatment. A positive response was obtained in 168 of 179 patients, leaving only 11 patients with no response at the onset of the first treatment. A normal bone scan showed no sign or symptom of prostate cancer in 28.3 percent of patients undergoing combination hormonal therapy, as compared to an average of only 4.6 percent in 5 recent studies in which patients were treated with monotherapy. The rate of complete positive responses achieved by combination hormonal therapy is increased by 6 times that of monotherapy. Another interesting finding is that only 6.1 percent of the patients did not show any positive response at the onset of the combination hormonal therapy, as compared to the average of 18 percent of the patients who did not respond to monotherapy. This is a 32.3 percent difference.

The duration of remission in those patients who were treated with combination hormonal therapy as compared to those receiving monotherapy was remarkable. At one year, it was 80.8 percent; at 2 years, it was 54 percent; and at 3 years, it was 38.9 percent. In a study by the European Organization for Research on the treatment of cancer, the percentages of patients still responding to treatment at 2 years were respectively 5 and 22 percent after monotherapy as compared to 54 percent with combination hormonal therapy.

The above data, which was obtained in the largest study ever performed using the objective criteria response of the U.S. National Prostate Cancer Project, indicates without a doubt that the use of combination hormonal therapy has a significant advantage over monotherapy. Combination hormonal therapy not only increases the rate of positive response at the onset of the treatment, but it also prolongs the duration of positive response as well as improves survival rates, as compared to all the other published studies using monotherapy. The decrease in the percentage of nonrespondents from 18 to 6.1 percent illustrates the significant advantage of combination hormonal therapy in both the quality of life and the survival rate for patients in which prostate cancer has spread to the bone at the onset of treatment.

Let's learn what some members of PAACT had to say to Ney about flutamide:

R.R., Bloomington, IN:

1992 looks a lot more promising than 1991 when I was diagnosed as having prostate cancer (D1) with a PSA count of 132.8.

After nearly one year on luprolide/flutamide my PSA count is now 0.1. I owe all of this to an article in *American Health Magazine* (December, 1990) written by an author after interviewing you. I have also talked to you on the phone and have received a lot of personal advice and help.

J.D., Bermuda Dunes, CA:

When I was diagnosed as having prostate cancer, stage D2 on March 2, 1992, I had a PSA of 1,856. I was placed on zoladex and flutamide therapy. By April 28, 1992, when I had my next PSA test, I was 1.0.

F.S., Thousand Oaks, CA:

Thank you for your many newsletters and solid advice on the phone. I feel fortunate to have learned about PAACT. Your experiences in the real world are far more valuable and objective than any information from urologists, radiation oncologists, oncologists, gastroenterologists, and others.

If I had to do it over again (20-20 hindsight), I would go with luprolide and flutamide only. I was on this treatment for six months immediately following diagnosis and never felt better. The tumor shrunk 25 percent and the urologist advised surgery. I opted for radiation and my energy level declined but I still play golf two or three times weekly. I am retired—very active, travel to Europe and other places two or three times a year.

As founder and president of International Post-graduate Medical Foundation, I conducted business with the world leaders in medicine, including heads of state, ministers of health, and prominent physicians. You are truly a breath of fresh air in the layman's world of medicine.

J.S., Portland, OR:

Five years, seven months since stage D prostate cancer diagnosis, and still going strong. Combination hormonal therapy does it!

Now that I have presented the multiple benefits of flutamide when used in combination with luprolide, as a prostate cancer patient you should understand that regardless of the stage of your disease, you should seriously consider being put on combination hormonal therapy immediately to downstage and debulk your cancerous tumor to make it more manageable for treatment. You should be aware that luprolide with flutamide is an effective agent for determining if your prostate cancer has spread to other parts of your body.

You should think twice before settling for an orchiectomy because you can be spared an operation and combination hormonal therapy can do a better job in shutting down the production of testosterone. You should request your physician to consider prescribing combination hormonal therapy if you have an advanced stage of prostate cancer to prolong your life; and you should demand that your doctor place you on flutamide and luprolide even if you have had a recurrence of your disease. Remember, some men have lived for ten years or more when placed on combination hormonal therapy even when the doctors had given them only months to live. Who knows, maybe you too can join the ten-year life time honor roll of receivers of flutamide and luprolide.

CHAPTER SEVEN

What You Should Know Before, During, and After Your Prostate Cancer Treatment

I believe that no one should ever go into any treatment without knowing what they will be putting their bodies through. Not only will you become knowledgeable about your treatment, but you will also gain a better understanding of the process, which will minimize surprises. I am reminded of the patient who underwent cryosurgery as his first choice of treatment and became upset because little was said of the postoperative pain between his penis and scrotum and the bruises and swelling of his penis. He was so upset that he wrote a column in *Cancer Communication* complaining about the whole situation. I do not know what he could have done about the swelling and pain other than to ask for a pain killer. At any rate, I think everyone should know the road they will travel when undergoing treatment for prostate cancer.

Although I discussed several treatments under each of the two pathways in Chapter Two, in this chapter I will discuss what patients should know before, during, and after treatment for the most common ones. Under the traditional pathway, this includes radical prostatectomy, external beam radiation, and bilateral orchiectomy, and under the nontraditional pathway, this includes seed implantation and cryosurgery. I have omitted other nontraditional treatments because they are not as popular as those indicated.

RADICAL PROSTATECTOMY

Radical prostatectomy is the surgical removal of the prostate gland and seminal vesicles in an attempt to cure prostate cancer. During this procedure, the bladder is brought down to the pelvis and the bladder neck is attached to the stump of the urethra at the point where the prostate gland was attached.

Preparation

During this phase of your treatment, your doctor will request that you donate time to save two or three pints of your own blood in the event of excessive bleeding during the operation. Because a radical prostatectomy is a very serious operation, I think it is prudent to advise you to prepare a living will as well as to give a relative or friend a durable power of attorney. You will also be asked to sign a health care proxy form. Although these may not be used, it is better to be safe than sorry. The mortality rate for this operation has been reported to be from 1 to 3 percent. By midnight on the night prior to surgery, a sign will be posted in your room or on your chart indicating that you cannot receive any food or drink until which time you recover fully from the effects of the anesthesia. This takes about 3 to 4 days after the operation. Be sure to contact your hospital insurance carrier to get your certification number to be admitted to the hospital. Call this number in to your hospital before the day of your admittance.

Preliminary Treatment

Prior to your treatment, you should consider whether or not to ask your urologist to consider putting you on combination hormonal therapy. In this debulking process, the stage of your disease may also be reclassified or downstaged. Look for a significant reduction in your PSA level.

Arrange Your Accommodations

Determine if you want a private or semiprivate room at the hospital and negotiate this with the hospital administration. Since you may be staying in the hospital for seven to ten days, make arrangements for television and telephone service.

Checking in to the Hospital

Before checking into the hospital, contact your hospital insurance carrier and see if you are required to give them prior notice. Your insurance company may require you to get a second opinion. Some hospital insurance carriers will not pay for any expenses for an operation unless you get the go ahead from them prior to the operation. In some hospitals, you may be requested to sign a consent to enable the surgeon to perform additional procedures if necessary, to allow another physician to assist your surgeon, and/or to sign a separate consent to cover risks and complications from anesthesia.

Once you have been checked into the hospital, a nurse will take your weight, blood pressure, pulse, and temperature. You will also be asked several medical-related questions, such as if you have any allergies, medication sensitivities, etc.

Antiseptic Cleaning

In preparation for the operation, you will be given enemas, as a bowel preparation. These procedures are performed to sterilize your intestines because your rectum may inadvertently be opened up during surgery. Sometimes your doctor may order a special antiseptic shower.

Introduction to the Anesthesiologist

Prior to the operation, your anesthesiologist will appear in your room to introduce himself or herself to you and to ask you a number of questions about your health. He or she may also explain the procedure that will be used to anesthetize you. A member of one of my support groups was rolled into the operating room only to be rolled out because the anesthesiologist would not anesthetize him since he had a previous heart condition.

Placement of Intravenous Drip

The nurse will insert a needle into your arm for emitting drugs that will help keep you anesthetized and relaxed during your operation.

Receiving a Sedative

Sometimes it is difficult for some patients who are going to be operated on to drop off to sleep the night proceeding the operation. Therefore, you may need to ask your doctor or the hospital to give you a sedative.

During the Surgery

On the morning of the operation, you will be brought to the waiting room. At this time, a nurse will review your plastic wristband to make certain you are the right patient for the operation. He or she will also check your chart. Once in the operating room, probably the first thing that will be done to you will be to give you a shot of a tranquilizer and another drug to prepare you for anesthesia. Sometimes, either in the waiting or the operating room, you will be asked if you have had anything to eat within the last twelve hours.

Once you are placed on the operating table, the anesthesiologist will prepare you for anesthesia by connecting you via electrodes to a heart monitor machine and various other equipment to watch your heartbeat, pulse, blood pressure, and body fluids. Your anesthesiologist will administer the anesthesia through an intravenous line through which the drug will travel to relax your muscles. This will make it easier for the surgeon to move them as he or she makes incisions through your lower abdomen to get to your prostate gland.

If you get a general anesthesia, the anesthesiologist will put a tube into your windpipe to control your breathing and to deliver the proper mixture of oxygen and anesthetic to your body. If you receive a spinal anesthetic, you will be hooked up to a monitoring machine and placed on an intravenous line. In order to make certain you do not feel any pain in the area of your incision, the anesthesiologist will administer to you a sedative and will inject anesthetics directly into your lower spine. Some doctors will also give you drugs to put you to sleep during the operation.

After two to five hours, depending on the difficulty of the surgery, your prostate gland and seminal vesicles will be removed. Then you will be wheeled into the recovery room. You may wake up in intensive care. One of the first things you will recognize after the anesthesia wears off is that your penis will have a bladder catheter inserted in it. The purpose of the catheter is to collect drainage so any blood and urine can come out without pooling in the pelvis. The urine that is collected is measured and used to provide a gauge as to how well your kidneys are functioning. The catheter and bottle will remain in you until there is no drainage or for up to three weeks after surgery.

In addition to the catheter, a tube will be sticking out of the site of the operation for a period of two to three days. A tube will be inserted into your nose through your stomach and connected to a suction machine so any accumulated fluid can be sucked out through the tube rather than left to cause your stomach to swell. This tube will be left in your nose for about four days until you are able to pass gas. Once this tube is removed, you will be able to eat a normal meal. Until that time, you will be fed intravenously.

After Surgery

After the operation, you may feel groggy and it may seem as though people are walking in slow motion. Rest assured that your anesthesiologist will visit you often to make certain there are no complications. You will also find yourself wearing special white socks to prevent clots in the veins that may gravitate toward the lungs. Keep your feet in motion as much as possible and lower your legs frequently to help prevent this condition.

The day after the operation, your doctor will most likely require you to walk around the hospital to prevent pneumonia and blood clots, and to help restore normal bowel functions. Your doctor may request that you take a deep breath at times to ascertain the probability of pneumonia. Some doctors may suggest that you avoid sitting during the first few days after the operation, and only to lie down or stand to avoid putting stress on your operation site.

Usually, you will remain in the hospital for seven days. You will leave the hospital with a catheter. Even after the catheter is removed, you will not be able to take full control of your urine and will leak urine for a few days and sometimes for months. As a result, your doctor may instruct you to wear pads inside your shorts. It will take you from three to six months or maybe years to perform your daily activities as you did prior to the operation.

Complications

What about complications associated with radical prostatectomy? These may fall into the following categories:

- Pain. Yes, you will experience some pain, but adjustable pain relieving machines are available in most modern hospitals that enable you to control it.

- Infection. Some researchers indicate that the rate of infection is as high as 5 percent. However, close monitoring by your doctor should prevent infection from occurring.

- Pneumonia. This is a serious complication, particularly for those who have prior lung problems. However, in most cases it is treatable.

- Rectal perforation. About one percent of patients who receive surgery have damage to the colon; however, usually this does not pose a serious problem.

- Death. Studies indicate that the death rate ranges from 1 to 3 percent. Do not be alarmed. There are several studies that show that the death rate is zero.

- Temporary incontinence. Studies indicate that the rate of temporary incontinence ranges from 1 to 4 percent. It has been reported that when the catheters are removed, one third of patients have already regained control of their urine, half regain control within one month, 25 percent by three months, and 95 percent within six months of surgery.

- Difficulty urinating. Some studies report that 6 to 12 percent of patients experience difficulty urinating because their surgery has led to narrowing of the neck of the bladder.

- Impotence. If you are Stage A1 or A2, the chances of restoring your sexual activity is 90 to 100 percent. If you are Stage B1 or B2, your chances of restoring your sexual activity are from 65 percent if you are between the ages of 55 and 59, and 55 percent if you are 60 to 69 years old.

Your doctor will schedule you to appear at his or her office in three months and then in six months. On each occasion, he or she will examine the incision, ask you a number of postoperative questions, and take a blood test to track your PSA level.

EXTERNAL BEAM RADIATION

External beam radiation is a process of bombarding and destroying prostate cancer cells by penetrating the prostate gland from the outside with high-energy protons. Today, a linear accelerator is usually used for this purpose. However, other machines are being introduced to perform this job without damaging noncancerous cells.

Preliminary Interview

During your initial interview with your radiation oncologist, he or she may require you to receive three to six months of combination therapy. Your medical records will be reviewed and discussed with you. You will be examined, and your weight, pulse rate, blood pressure, and heart rate will be determined. You will also receive a blood test to ascertain a current PSA level.

Your radiation oncologist will give you a date to return to his or her office after you complete your combination hormonal treatment to begin the next phase. Often during this interview, you will also be introduced to the procedural steps for performing radiation treatment, how much radiation treatment, and other related particulars.

Special Tests

When your radiation oncologist is satisfied that you are ready to begin your radiation treatment, you will be requested to eat nothing the night before the day on which you will undergo special tests for pinpointing your treatment site. In a process called simulation, you will be requested to lie on a table while your radiation oncologist inserts a foley catheter into your penis to insert a fluid into your bladder in order to illuminate your prostate gland. A computer is programmed with information gathered in the CT scan in order to define the treatment points. The foley catheter is slightly painful and discomforting.

A radiation oncologist will mark your treatment points on the skin of your pubic area with tiny dots of colored, semipermanent ink to define the treatment site. Once your simulation is completed, a final decision is made as to how much radiation will be needed for your treatment, how it will be delivered, and how many treatments you should have. This particular procedure should take from two to three hours. It is done with the help of a radiation physicist.

Treatment

You and your radiation oncologist will agree to a schedule for your treatments. You will receive external beam radiation therapy five days per week for six to seven weeks with each treatment lasting from three to five minutes. Each week of your treatment, a nurse will track your weight, heart beat, and blood pressure. In addition, your doctor will also examine you weekly to follow your progress, checking your response to the treatment and overall health.

Prior to any radiation treatment, you will be required to change into a hospital gown. Sometimes when undergoing radiation treatment, a special shield is placed around certain parts of your body to help protect them from damage. Once on the treatment table, you will be requested to remain absolutely still to confine your radiation treatment to the treatment site. Your therapist will leave the treatment room before the machine is turned on. Although you may feel alone, your therapist is able to see you either on a television monitor or through a window in the control room.

During your treatment, your radiation oncologist may perform another simulation check to further readjust the radiation beam to cover a greater area, which may be outside your prostate gland. On the last day of your treatment or soon thereafter, your radiation oncologist will order another blood test, examine you, and ask you if there are any problems with your treatment. He or she will also request that you appear in his or her office again in three and six months to reexamine you and take another blood test to determine if any cancer has been left in your prostate gland.

Complications

What about complications associated with external beam radiation? Although they may be unpleasant, they usually are not serious if your hospital uses updated equipment, such as the linear accelerator. Your complications may consist of the following:

- Diarrhea. Some patients undergoing external beam radiation treatment complain of diarrhea after a certain number of treatments. This was not a problem for me.

- Urination frequency. Any urination frequency experienced prior to treatment should diminish as a result of tumor shrinkage due to the radiation and combination hormonal therapy if you were also administered this treatment. Although I am not going to the bathroom as often as I did prior to the operation, I still go from one to two times per night.

- Impotency. Studies seem to suggest that this depends on how potent you were prior to radiation treatment. If you had a strong erection prior to the treatment, the probability is high that you will remain potent. If on the other hand your erection was weak prior to treatment, it will most likely be weaker after treatment. Some studies indicate impotency rate may be as high as 50 percent. It can take several months to recover potency after combination hormonal therapy and radiation treatment.

- Flatulence. Some patients indicated that they did not experience this complication as a serious problem. I found this to be a problem during and after my radiation treatment. Almost daily, I had several incidents of "passing gas," and at times, it was very embarrassing. Perhaps the most difficult problem I experienced were incidents in which I thought I would pass gas and actually moved my bowels.

- Painful urination may be a problem.

BILATERAL ORCHIECTOMY

During Surgery

Bilateral orchiectomy is removal of the testicles to halt the production of testosterone. An anesthesiologist will introduce himself or herself to you and ask you a number of questions to determine if you have a heart condition, are allergic to any medication, and a number of other questions. He or she will give you either a local or general anesthetic.

Your operating doctor will most likely make a small incision, no more than one to two inches long in the middle portion of the lower part of your scrotum (between the two testes) and remove both of your testes. Some urologists will make a small incision on each side of your scrotum and remove the respective testes. Although this operation can be done on an outpatient basis, some doctors might request you to stay in the hospital for one or two days following surgery.

After Surgery

Because the scrotum contains few pain fibers, you should experience very little discomfort. Your incision(s) should heal fairly rapidly.

Complications

Complications associated with bilateral orchiectomy are as follows:

- It cannot be reversed if an absolute cure is found for prostate cancer.
- Some men suffer psychologically because of the removal of the testes.
- Breast tenderness occurs in some patients.
- Some patients complain of hot flashes.
- Other side effects may include chronic infection and bleeding.

SEED IMPLANTATION

I-125 seed implantation is a form of brachytherapy whereby Iodine-125 seeds are permanently implanted directly in the middle of the prostate cancer where they give off low-level radiation continuously for approximately one year. As stated in a previous chapter, palladium is also used in implants.

Seed implantation is normally done as an outpatient procedure and takes about one hour to perform. The patient usually leaves the hospital the same day as the implant procedure and resumes normal activities within several days. However, if you have an enlarged prostate gland, your physician should place you on combination hormonal therapy for 3 to 6 months prior to seed implantation to debulk your prostate gland to make it more manageable for treatment.

Three Weeks Prior to the Implant

A volume study, to determine the location and size of the cancer, will usually be performed. Using a TRUS unit, the urologist will locate your prostate and a computer will take several pictures showing the location and size of the cancer. These pictures will assist the medical physicist to determine the number of iodine seeds needed to treat the prostate and exactly where they should be placed.

One Week Prior to the Implant

You will have blood tests done and possibly an electrocardiogram (EKG) and chest X-ray. Your doctor will determine which tests are necessary. The test results are used to inform the anesthesiologist of your ability to tolerate anesthesia.

One to Two Days Prior to the Implant

One to two days before the implant, you will be given specific instructions regarding diet and enemas. The enema will help remove fecal material from your lower bowel and rectum so that the ultrasound image of your prostate will be clear.

On the Day of the Implant

The radioactive seed implant procedure is performed in the operating room and lasts about 45 minutes to 1 hour. You will probably receive spinal anesthesia, leaving you numb from the waist down. You may also receive medication through an intravenous (IV) line, which will make you feel drowsy. An ultrasound probe will be inserted into the rectum to image the prostate on a television monitor. The seeds, usually about 50 to 80 in number, are then inserted into the prostate with needles, through the skin between the scrotum and the rectum and, with the TRUS device, are guided with pinpoint accuracy directly to the tumor sites. At the end of the procedure, a catheter is temporarily placed in your bladder to drain urine.

After the Implant

After the implant, you will go to a recovery room for about two hours, until you have regained feeling in your legs. While in the recovery room, you will have an ice bag placed between your legs to help reduce swelling of the implant area. The urinary catheter is usually removed when you have regained feeling in your legs. Occasionally, the catheter is left in overnight. Since the seed implant is generally an outpatient procedure, you can go home after you have recovered from the anesthesia. Because you may feel a little weak, it is recommended that you do not drive for at least twelve hours. You may wish to resume eating and have visitors, but you should avoid heavy lifting or strenuous physical activity for the first two days you are home. After that, you will probably be ready to return to your normal activity level.

Complications

Some complications are associated with I-125 seed implantation. These fall into the following categories:

- Seed implantation may hide the efficiency of subsequent treatment.

- Incontinence occurs in less than 5 percent of patients who have not had prior surgery.

- Impotence occurs in less than 15 percent of patients under the age of 70. For patients over the age of 70, impotence occurs more often.

- There is no information yet on the effectiveness of the implant treatment after ten years. While the current clinical data show good results throughout the first five years, younger men are advised to more strongly consider radical prostatectomy or external beam radiation.

- It is very common to experience problems with urination after seed implantation. These symptoms will gradually decrease after six to twelve months.

CRYOSURGERY

Cryosurgery is a procedure of destroying cancerous cells in the prostate gland through freezing it with liquid nitrogen at a temperature of -196°C using a transrectal ultrasound machine to monitor the freezing process.

Preliminary Treatment

Similarly to radical prostatectomy, you may be administered combination hormonal therapy for three to six months to debulk and downstage your disease. Prior to being wheeled to the operating room, you may also get a dose of an antibiotic as added protection against infection.

Pre-Admission Testing

You will undergo several tests before you are admitted to the hospital. You will get a blood test for a new PSA level, several other blood tests, and possibly an MRI, including transrectal MRI. You will also undergo the regular routine tests, such as blood pressure, heart rate, pulse, and weight. The nurse will determine if you brought all the required blood test results, X-ray reports, bone scans, MRIs, and biopsies. The intent of these tests is to determine if you have any serious medical problems that might need to be treated. You will also be examined by either your surgeon or another physician. Since cryosurgery is an investigative treatment, you will have to sign a consent form.

Placement of Intravenous Drip

A nurse will insert the needle for intravenous antibiotics into your arm, take your vital signs, and give you a tablet to help you avoid nausea after the anesthesia wears off so you can eat.

Introduction to Your Anesthesiologist

Once you are wheeled into the operation, and sometimes before the operation, your anesthesiologist will introduce himself or herself to you and ask if you are allergic to any drugs and if you have had any experience with anesthesia. The procedure for anesthetizing will be explained and drugs introduced by the intravenous drip will begin to take effect. A tube will be put into your windpipe to control your breathing and to deliver the proper mixture of oxygen and anesthesia to your body. A mask will be placed over your face and your anesthesiologist will closely monitor you through the various indicators on the machine.

During Surgery

With you anesthetized, your doctors will use ultrasound image guidance to insert five needles into your prostate gland. These needles are passed through the area between your anus and scrotum. The ultrasound allows your doctors to monitor the effect of the freezing substance that is passed through the needles. A catheter will be put in your penis to keep the urethra warm so it will not freeze during the procedure.

After Surgery

During the night after the operation, a nurse will visit you to take your vital signs. One day after surgery you will be sched uled for another MRI and a transrectal MRI. Your doctor will check you out of the hospital with the catheter still in you. Your doctor will advise you when to remove the catheter, inform you of what you can expect postsurgery, and request that you see him or her every three months for a period of two years.

Complications

What complications are you likely to experience with cryosurgery? They fall into the following categories:

- Pain. Some pain will be experienced from your anus to your scrotum. Your penis will be swollen. In addition, you may also experience some discomfort from the tube placed in your windpip⌐. However, pain relief pills should help.

- Impotency. Up to 40 percent of patients who were potent prior to surgery remained potent shortly thereafter. Others resume their potency eventually. However, the final percentage is not known at this time.

- Leakage of urine. If you are experiencing this side effect, it may heal spontaneously with the use of a urinary catheter; however, minor surgery is sometimes necessary.

- Repeat freeze. If the first freezing does not destroy all the cancerous cells, you may have to be refrozen a second or third time.

STANDARD OFFICE PROCEDURE
REGARDLESS OF TREATMENT TYPE

Whether you are going to your doctor's office after radical prostatectomy, radiation therapy, or combination hormonal treatment, your periodic visits should include the following:

- Digital rectal examination

- PSA blood test

- Periodic CT and bone scan to make certain there are no signs of residual cancer

After your treatment for prostate cancer, you (and I emphasize *you*) should remain alert to a recurrence of cancer. By closely monitoring your condition, you may be able to detect any remaining cancer or recurrence of cancer.

Some of the steps cited in this chapter may or may not be included in the treatment delivered to you. On the other hand, other steps peculiar to your physician may be included or may vary from the standard treatment. This usually occurs because of the unique experience of your physicians. Once you have decided on a treatment, familiarize yourself with the procedure described in this chapter and query your doctor as to how closely he or she will follow it.

CHAPTER EIGHT

Questions and Answers About Prostate Cancer

I decided to write this chapter to respond to questions that were not covered previously. These questions were raised during the numerous meetings of my prostate support groups and in the multitude of books and professional articles I read. Some of the questions were also given to me by wives, children, and friends who had loved ones suffering from prostate cancer, as well as questions I thought would be of interest to the general public. From time to time, I am called upon by colleagues to respond to queries they have in regard to diagnosis and treatment. I am careful not to prescribe, but to relate the research and findings. I have included these questions, also.

On several occasions, I have accompanied prostate cancer patients to their physicians for support and guidance. Usually, I attend examination rooms with the doctor and patient and questions are asked of the physicians by me and the patient. I have also included these questions. Afterward, the patients ask for clarification regarding something the doctor said. These questions are included, as well.

QUESTION: What is my risk of prostate cancer?

ANSWER: I am focussing on two major factors, ethnic groups and race and genetic factors. However, there are several others, such as diet, sexual activity, marital status, viral factors, suppressor gene mutations, environmental factors, etc.

There are huge differences in the incidence of prostate cancer between ethnic groups and geographic locations. Consider the following statistics:

Location	Incidence of prostate cancer per 100,000 males[2]
USA, California, Alameda County, blacks	100.2
USA, Michigan, Detroit, blacks	73.2
USA, Georgia, Atlanta, whites	51.9
Sweden	44.4
USA, Hawaii, Hawaiian	42.5
USA, Michigan, Detroit, whites	41.4
New Zealand, Maori	39.8
Australia, South Australia	39.6
Norway	38.9
USA, Hawaii, Japanese	35.9
Germany, Saarland.	32.9
New Zealand, Non-Maori.	30.7
Jamaica, Kingston and St. Andrew	28.6
Finland.	27.2
USA, California, Los Angeles County, Chinese	26.6
France, Doubs.	25.7
Denmark.	23.6
UK, Scotland, North-East	23.4
Italy, Varese	22.8
USA, California, Los Angeles County, Japanese.	21.5
Spain, Zaragoza	20.7
Cuba	19.9
UK, England and Wales, Mersey region.	18.1
Germany, Dresden	18.1
Spain, Navarra.	17.6
Yugoslavia, Slovenia	15.8
Israel, Jews.	15.5
Poland, Warsaw	14.6
Japan, Nagasaki	10.2
Romania, County Cluj.	9.7
Czechoslovakia, Western Slovakia	8.1

Singapore, Malay 7.2
India, Bombay 6.8
Ho.. g Kong 5.1
Singapore, Chinese 4.8
Africa, Senegal, Dakar 4.23

The above statistics indicate that the highest incidence of prostate cancer is in the United States and Scandinavia. The lowest rate occurs in Asia. Intermediate rates are in England, France, and Italy. In the United States, there are some unique differences. For example, African Americans who live in Detroit have nearly double the rate than that for whites living in the same city. Another interesting feature about the statistics is that prosperity seems to make very little difference when considering blacks and whites in Detroit. Further, while African Americans have the highest incidence of prostate cancer in the world, Africans in Senegal, Dakar, have the lowest.

When we consider the accumulated data of records of more than 8,000 patients in the PAACT database, the following table indicates the risk of getting prostate cancer considering the genetic factors:

No family history of cancer . . . . 1 in 9   (11.2%)
Family history of cancer other than prostate . . . . . 2 in 9   (18.9%)
Both parents with cancer other than prostate . . . . 2 in 5   (42.6%)
Father had prostate cancer, mother other cancer . 1 in 2   (53.1%)
Father and uncle had prostate cancer . . . . 3 in 5   (61.7%)
Grandfather, father and uncle(s)
had prostate cancer . . . . 4 in 5   (86.3%)

The above chart indicates that prostate cancer tends to be hereditary. If your father had prostate cancer and your mother had some form of cancer, there is a fifty-fifty chance that you will suffer from the disease. However, the probability that you will get prostate cancer increases depending on the number of family members on your father's side who had cancer.

QUESTION: What are some gold standards for either the diagnosis or treatment for prostate cancer?

ANSWER: These so-called gold standards do not mean that they are right for you. They are only standards that doctors have given to these treatments for prostate cancer. These gold standards are as follows:

- PAACT mentions that combination hormo⌐ ⌐erapy is the gold standard for downstaging and debulking of all stages of prostate cancer, although some physicians doubt this claim.

- Radical prostatectomy is the gold standard for the treatment of prostate cancer.

- Bilateral orchiectomy remains the gold standard for shutting down the production of testosterone or for the initial treatment of advanced prostate cancer, although some researchers dispute this.

QUESTION: What are some of the reasons that some doctors provide combination hormonal therapy as an immediate treatment to patients with advanced prostate cancer?

ANSWER: There are several. These are as follows:

- To markedly improve survival.

- To downstage the disease.

- To debulk the disease and to make it more manageable.

- To treat a tumor while it is smaller rather than when it is large to prevent complication from uncontrolled tumor growth.

- To try to prevent or delay metastatic spread.

QUESTION: In addition to being of some value in the detection of prostate cancer, is there another value for performing a bloodtest for determining a patient's PSA level?

ANSWER: Yes. In fact, it appears that the most useful value in determining a patient's PSA level is after either a radical prostatectomy, radiation therapy, or some other treatment. If both the benign and malignant prostatic tissue have been removed, or if the cancer cells in the prostate gland have been destroyed by either radiation, freezing, heating, etc., a post-PSA level should be nil. On the other hand, a detectable trend in the PSA is usually indicative of remaining cancer cells. Two studies indicate that those patients who have an elevated PSA level between 3 and 4 months after treatment have a 100 percent chance of a recurrence of the disease. However, my radiation oncologist has indicated to me that an accurate PSA level can only be determined after 6 months of treatment when a base point is established. Subsequently, PSA blood tests should be taken every 3 months for a period of 1 year. After 1 year, the PSA can be taken every 6 to 12 months. During this period, the physician should be alert to a trend in an elevated PSA, which may signal a progression or recurrence of prostate cancer.

QUESTION: I am an African American. My father and my two brothers had prostate cancer. Would I decrease my chances of getting prostate cancer if I get a radical prostatectomy prior to being diagnosed with the disease?

ANSWER: I would think so. However, you may be the only male of the family who does not get prostate cancer. Another thing you must consider is what new treatments may be available in the future that may be an improvement over existing treatments. The question is, should you get a serious operation like a radical prostatectomy if you do not need one?

QUESTION: What are some common mistakes made by some physicians in either the diagnosis or treatment of prostate cancer?

ANSWER: Based on my experience and interaction with physicians and colleagues in my two prostate cancer support groups, the common mistakes are as follows:

- Intimidating prostate cancer victims to undergo immediate treatment before adequately explaining the various available treatments.

- Failing to perform all of the necessary tests to make an accurate assessment of prostate cancer patients' stage.

- Failing to divulge a prostate cancer patients' PSA level, Gleason grade, or stage.

- Withholding information from patients about the side effects of various treatments.

- Failing to remain abreast of recent research, new medical technology, new procedures, and improved treatments.

- Failing to perform an adequate (at least six) number of punctures during a biopsy.

- Failing to use combination hormonal therapy to shrink an enlarged prostate gland in order to make it more manageable for treatment.

- Failing to conduct a digital rectal examination and/or PSA blood test during an annual physical examination.

- Understaging prostate cancer patients.

- Failing to perform the DNA ploidy analysis in an effort to determine if a patient's prostate cancer is slow growing.

- Failing to develop a watchful waiting criteria and failing to consider this option before proceeding with either radical prostatectomy or external beam radiation.

- Failing to advise patients as to where they can go to receive radiation treatment from a hospital that has the latest medical technology.

- Failing to give prostate cancer patients a copy of their medical records.

- Maintaining a certain bias for specific treatments based on limited knowledge of research, ignorance, and/or lack of experience with other treatments.

- Giving prostate cancer patients incorrect information or withholding information.

- Failing to properly prescribe medication to their patients. (Many physicians indicate to their patients to take "two capsules of flutamide three times daily," when it should be "two capsules every eight hours.")

QUESTION: What are some common mistakes made by prostate cancer victims when diagnosed with the disease?

ANSWER: The following are mistakes that I have made or were committed by colleagues in my prostate cancer support groups:

- Failing to become fortified with sufficient knowledge about prostate cancer prior to accepting a specific treatment.

- Relying only on the traditional pathway to decide on a treatment for prostate cancer, rather than considering both traditional and nontraditional pathways.

- Continuing to remain under the care of a physician who has used outmoded procedures; given erroneous information; failed to divulge side effects of various treatments; and is not current with the latest research on prostate cancer.

- Failing to ask for a digital rectal examination and PSA blood test during annual physical examinations.

- Failing to ask their physicians about their PSA level, Gleason scores, grade, and stage.

- Failing to consider watchful waiting as an option prior to treatment.

- Failing to join a prostate cancer support group, or joining after treatment rather than prior to treatment.

- Allowing physicians to intimidate them into undergoing treatment for prostate cancer without adequate exploration of the disease.

- Gaining knowledge about a specific treatment not known to the physician and failing to request him or her to investigate it to determine if it should be prescribed by the patient. An excellent example is the use of combination hormonal therapy to debulk an enlarged prostate prior to radical prostatectomy.

- Relying on diet alone to treat a recurrence of prostate cancer rather than attempting to arrest the disease using a holistic approach, which also includes treatment under the traditional and/or nontraditional pathway.

- Failing to track the PSA level every three months for a period of one year, beginning six months after the treatment, and gradually extending the tracking period.

- Remaining with an insensitive physician who does not have adequate time to spend with his or her patients to respond to their needs for information and/or concerns.

- Failing to reschedule himself for either another PSA blood test or biopsy within 3 or 4 months when an initial biopsy failed to detec the prostate cancer.

QUESTION: Why is combination hormonal therapy not used as a treatment for prostate cancer?

ANSWER: Combination hormonal therapy shuts down the body system to produce testosterone, which is needed by cancer cells to grow. However, all cancer cells do not need testosterone to grow. The following are the three kinds of cancer cells that can determine what type of treatment you should receive:

- Those that depend on testosterone to nourish prostate cancer cells.

- Those that are not totally dependent on testosterone, but receive some impetus from it.

- Those cancer cells that can grow and flourish without testosterone.

In prostate cancer, approximately 80 to 90 percent of the cells are linked in one way or another to testosterone. These cells are identified as hormone sensitive. The other 10 to 20 percent of the cells are hormone insensitive. They are sort of outlaws that do not depend on androgens to destroy the prostate. As a result, the outlaws overcome any hormonal treatment and pursue a course of human destruction, unless another defense is instituted that is fatal to these outlaw cells.

QUESTION: When is a patient deemed to be cured of prostate cancer?

ANSWER: Not everybody can be cured of prostate cancer. If you are Stage A or B, the chances of being cured of the disease are high. If you are Stage C1, depending on the spread of the disease, you may be cured. On the other hand, if you are Stage C2, C3, D0, D1, D2, or D3, the probability of a cure is remote. Usually, when the doctor indicates a cure, it means that there is no detectable sign of cancer and the patient has the same expectancy as if he never had cancer.

I believe this is a falsehood. A person may have been treated with combination hormonal therapy and have no signs of cancer present, like Lloyd Ney, and still be considered not cured. Perhaps an improved definition of the term cure would involve a time frame, such as, "when there is no evidence of the cancer for ten years." Once again, we have a problem. Ney has been cleared of prostate cancer for a number of years and will be approaching ten years soon. However, he will not be considered cured in the eyes of many doctors. I for one do not know if a person is ever cured of prostate cancer. There have been occasions in which prostate cancer patients have had their cancer confined to the prostate gland, which was verified through a radical prostatectomy and have been announced as cured, and then several years thereafter, the disease had metastasized elsewhere in the body. This occurred because of the microscopic nature of some prostate cancer cells that cannot be detected with the current level of our medical technology.

QUESTION: Once a treatment recommendation is made by my doctor, should I get a second and even a third opinion?

ANSWER There is nothing more important than your life. Therefore, you should never be satisfied with one professional opinion. I personally had three urologists, four radiation oncologists, and one oncologist give me their professional opinion about the diagnosis and treatment of my prostate cancer.

QUESTION: When my doctor examined my lymph nodes, it was found that there was no evidence of tumor involvement. Does this mean that my cancer has not spread beyond my prostate gland?

ANSWER: No, because the cancer may have already spread to the bones, but the changes in the bones occurred too early to be detected on the bone scan. Another reason why your lymph nodes may seem to be free of the spread of the disease is because when the lymph nodes are removed and examined by the pathologist, he or she only examines a random sampling of those lymph nodes where there is a high probability of a spread of cancer.

QUESTION: What treatment is recommended for a patient who is experiencing bone pain due to prostate cancer?

ANSWER: Combination hormonal therapy with the possible addition of localized external beam radiation therapy has been found to be effective. In addition, numerous radioisotopes and biphosphonates have been effective in varying degrees. You and your physicians should consider one of these: clodronate, etidronate, samarium, strontium-89, iridium, sandostatin, samatuline, somatostatin, and lovastatin.

QUESTION: Is it possible for a patient to opt for radiation therapy, and if that fails, to have his prostate removed?

ANSWER: Yes, it is possible, but it is certainly not recommended. True, radiation therapy would kill the cancerous cells, but it also has an impact on healthy cells. If the radiation therapy fails and you have your prostate removed, you probably will experience some serious postoperative side effects. Research has shown that some patients who have had radiation after surgery do have a slightly increased risk of developing urinary problems, experiencing swelling of the legs, and suffering from injury to the rectum and other organs. If you had radical prostatectomy first, followed by external beam radiation, you have lessened your chances of being adversely affected by the complications. Radiation therapy would be a sound alternative if it has been determined that some cancerous cells still remain in your body. The side effects associated with using radiation after surgery are far less severe than those associated with surgery performed after radiation. Recently, PAACT has opposed this treatment.

QUESTION: What is the best time for me to get my treatment after I have been diagnosed with prostate cancer?

ANSWER: This depends on whether or not you asked to be put on combination hormonal therapy. If you requested combination hormonal therapy as a prior treatment, then the period is from three to six months for the purpose of debulking the volume of your prostate gland and downstaging your disease. If you have not opted for combination hormonal therapy, Leonard G. Gomella, author of *Recovering From Prostate Cancer* (Harper Paperbooks, New York: 1993), writes, "almost half a dozen studies suggest that if you delay more than three months between the time your cancer has been diagnosed and the time you begin therapy, you are playing a dangerous game of diminishing your chances of beating the disease."

QUESTION: What is meant by a double-blind clinical trial?

ANSWER: Usually, a double-blind study is conducted in a clinical trial when a group of patients is divided into two groups to determine the value of an experiment. One group receives the experimental treatment, while the other group receives a placebo. Neither group is aware of what they are receiving and neither are their physicians.

QUESTION: What is the disadvantage of a double-blind study?

ANSWER: If the experiment works, only some of the members will have benefited from the experiment, while some of the members of the placebo group may have died during the course of the experiment.

QUESTION: Can you give me some idea as to how it feels to the doctor when he or she touches a normal prostate compared to a malignant prostate gland?

ANSWER: Yes. Place your index finger at the tip of your nose and press gently. This is what a normal prostate feels like. Now, make a fist of your left hand and place your right index finger on your first left knuckle. A similar hard feeling on your prostate may indicate cancer of the prostate. In addition, a slightly raised or lumpy area on the otherwise smooth and spongy or soft surface of the prostate gland could also signal a cancerous growth.

QUESTION: Should the digital rectal examination be performed before or after the PSA blood test?

ANSWER: Some doctors maintain that by stimulating the rectum with a digital rectal examination, the PSA blood level is raised, producing a false indication of cancer. Therefore, those doctors maintain that the digital rectal examination should be performed after the PSA blood test. A study by the Prostate Cancer Education Council disproved this theory by showing that PSA blood levels were not any higher either prior to or after the digital rectal examination.

QUESTION: I was under the impression that radical prostatectomy is only for patients who are Stage A or B; however, I was recently informed that some Stage D1 patients are also candidates for this treatment. Is this true?

ANSWER: True, radical prostatectomy is usually reserved for prostate cancer patients who are stage A or B. However, there appears to be some evidence that men who have been Stage D1 that involved microscopic lymph nodes metastasis may benefit from radical prostatectomy in an effort to control the core of the disease. Some Stage D1 patients who have been treated with radical prostatectomy followed by combination hormonal therapy have had a biological change in their bodies resulting in a doubling of the median survival time when compared to those who have not had the tumor removed through surgery. Recently, PAACT has opposed this treatment.

QUESTION: What can I do to determine if my lymph nodes have been invaded by cancer prior to undergoing a radical prostatectomy and pelvic examination?

ANSWER: Some physicians are beginning to use a rectal coil MRI to image the lymph nodes for examination purposes. If there appears to be no evidence of cancer in the lymph nodes, they will follow this examination with a laparoscopic lymph node dissection of the remaining lymph nodes.

As I stated previously, until I wrote this book, I did not know of these tests. If I had, I certainly would have added these to the others I chose for myself. None of my doctors advised me of these tests. I hope you give serious consideration to them and insist that your doctor perform them. It may be the final proof that your disease has not spread beyond your prostate gland.

QUESTION: After treatment, what is the probability that I will be alive in five years?

ANSWER: The five-year number is important because it is used by many practitioners as a threshold. If you live past five years after treatment, your chances of living a full life greatly improve. The overall survival rates for each stage are as follows:

Stage A: The chances of surviving after your diagnosis and treatment and that you will live a full life if you are a Stage A patient is nearly 100 percent.

Stage B: If you are a Stage B patient, there is an 85 percent probability that you will live a full life after diagnosis and treatment. In fact, the American Cancer Society, in its 1992 *Cancer Facts and Figures Report*, maintains that the five-year survival rate for victims of prostate cancer if your cancer is confined to the prostate gland is nearly 90 percent. However, a ten- and fifteen-year survival rate is more important than five-year survival since prostate cancer is generally slow growing.

Stage C: If you are a Stage C patient, the chances of your surviving after the fifth year if your disease has spread to areas near your prostate is 70 percent.

Stage D: When you get to Stage D, your survival seems gloomy. When your prostate cancer has reached other areas of your body such as your bones, kidneys, lungs, etc., your five-year survival rate is only about 30 percent. I believe this figure will change in the future because of combination hormonal therapy. I am not saying that once you are diagnosed as a Stage D patient and are treated with combination hormonal therapy, that the five-year survival period for you is certain. I am saying that this therapy works for some Stage D patients. It may not necessarily work for you, but let us be hopeful.

QUESTION: I know that the use of flutamide affects a person's ability to have sex. Does chemotherapy also affect this same ability?

ANSWER: Chemotherapy, the use of drugs or medication to treat prostate cancer, generally does not affect the ability to have or the desire for sex. Some men find that the stress of the disease or their treatment schedule makes them feel more tired than usual and therefore, their sexual activity is infrequent.

QUESTION: What is an ideal patient for a radical prostatectomy?

ANSWER: If the disease has been confined to the prostate, the person is under the age of 70, the Gleason score is 4 or less, the PSA level is under 10 ng/ml, and the person is generally in good health. However, this is not an ironclad rule.

QUESTION: Can zinc prevent or treat prostate cancer?

ANSWER: Researchers have not found that zinc will prevent prostate cancer or that it is a viable treatment. William Fair, M.D., a urologist at Memorial Sloan-Kettering Cancer Center in New York City, has conducted a long-term study of zinc and the prostate gland. He maintains that zinc may be important in the prevention of prostate cancer. He goes on to say that the prostate cannot pick up and utilize zinc when it is consumed orally. He further states that even when zinc is absorbed by the bloodstream, the prostate is unable to utilize the zinc. On the other hand, Dr. Fair says that tests have proven that the zinc levels are definitely lower in men with prostate cancer. He does not know if this is because of the cancer attacking the prostate or if the cancer gets a foothold on the prostate because the zinc level is low.

Some experts say that zinc can be used as an effective method for preventing prostate problems. This theory seems to be growing in this country. The only way I can respond to this question is to say that zinc is necessary for a healthy and properly functioning prostate gland. Many more questions remain, such as how does the prostate absorb and utilize whatever zinc it needs? Therefore, in closing my response to this question, I can only say that some doctors are prescribing long-term use of zinc sulphate by mouth as a means to prevent and treat certain kinds of prostate problems. However, a dear friend of mine who has been taking zinc tablets for years has recently been diagnosed with prostate cancer.

QUESTION: If an ultrasound probe is an effective means to detect prostate cancer, why shouldn't I request that my doctor use this detection method instead of the digital rectal examination?

ANSWER: This sounds like good advice to me, particularly because the finger can only detect tumors over a certain size and only on a limited portion of the prostate, whereas the ultrasound probe can pick up cancer as small as 5 mm in diameter (under a quarter inch). On the other hand, it is difficult to distinguish on the ultrasound scan between certain types of prostate disease and prostate cancer. I guess we are back to the good old digital rectal examination.

QUESTION: What is meant by salvage therapy?

ANSWER: When the original treatment for prostate cancer fails or is not certain to have produced a complete cure, another treatment is performed to kill the remaining cancer cells or tumor. For example, often external beam radiation is used as a salvage treatment for radical prostatectomy if marginal disease is suspected. It should be understood that not all treatments can be used as salvage therapy without serious complications; i.e., utilizing brachytherapy as a salvage therapy following external beam radiation.

QUESTION: I am aware that PAACT has a computerized information database from which I can retrieve information about certain subjects related to prostate cancer. Is there another source from which I can get information on prostate cancer?

ANSWER: Yes, the National Cancer Institute has developed Physician's Data Query (PDQ), a computerized database designed to give doctors quick and easy access to the latest treatment information on prostate cancer, description of clinical trials that are available for patients with prostate cancer, and names of organizations and doctors involved in prostate cancer. Patients can use the PDQ by calling 1-800-4-CANCER.

QUESTION: My doctor suspects that my prostate cancer has spread to other organs of my body and has recommended that I get an MRI as opposed to a CT scan. What are the advantages and disadvantages of an MRI over a CT scan?

ANSWER: A major advantage of the MRI over the CT scan is its ability to show an image in three complementary planes. Therefore, the image is made sharper. The disadvantages are it is more costly and confining. Therefore, if you suffer from claustrophobia, you may have a problem with the technology. More recently, this problem has been satisfied by using an open space machine rather than a capsule. However, if your physician suggests that your disease has spread to other organs of your body, he or she should also consider using the rectal coil MRI to determine if your disease has spread to your lymph nodes.

QUESTION: I understand that radiation works to destroy prostate cancer cells over a period of time, not instantly. Is there any truth to this statement?

ANSWER: A survey of 30 patients treated with radiation showed that 6 months after radiation treatment, 66 percent of men still had traces of cancer. However, 12 months after treatment, 31 percent still had cancer cells. And after 3.5 years had passed, cancer was seen in 19 percent of the patients. This gradual reduction of cancer cells in the prostate means that radiation does not kill a cancer cell as much as it cripples its ability to reproduce itself.

QUESTION: Why is it that my doctor is still giving me a digital rectal examination when my prostate gland has been removed through surgery?

ANSWER: Even though your prostate gland has been surgically removed, your physician should examine the area in which your prostate was once located to feel for firm or irregular tissue. Even though this digital rectal examination may not reveal a suspicion of recurrence of prostate cancer, from time to time your physician should also perform a prostate specific antigen (PSA) blood test to determine your PSA level. If there is a steady rise in your PSA level, a biopsy should subsequently be performed.

QUESTION: Who are some of the pioneers in the diagnosis and treatment of prostate cancer?

ANSWER: Richard J. Ablin, Ph.D., of Innapharma, Inc. in Suffern, New York is one of the leading scientists responsible for identifying prostatic specific antigen.

John Blasko, M.D., a radiation oncologist at the Northwest Tumor Institute in Seattle, Washington, is the lead physician to maximize the efficiency of I-125 seed implantation, an effective alternative treatment for prostate cancer.

Patrick Walsh, M.D., a urologist at John Hopkins University, is the physician that perfected the nerve-sparing surgical treatment for prostate cancer to minimize the side effect of impotency.

Fernand Labrie, M.D., of Laval University of Quebec, Canada developed combination hormonal therapy, which is used to block androgens at the adrenal glands.

Fred Lee, M.D., is a radiation oncologist, head of the department at the Crittenton Hospital in Rochester, Michigan and the world's leading authority in observation and interpretation of transrectal ultrasound cryosurgery.

Willet Whitmore, M.D., a retired urologist, is a leading proponent in this country of the watchful waiting and devised the criteria for classifying prostate cancer into stages A, B, C, and D according to tumor size, prevalence, and metastatic stage.

Thomas Stamey, M.D., and John McNeal, M.D., of the Stanford Medical School are responsible for perfecting the whole mount theory, which maintains that tumor size alone is a fair gauge of malignancy, for as cancer cells divide, they undergo a series of mutations that increase their oppressive behavior, which may lead them to escape from the prostate gland.

Malcolm Bagshaw, Ph.D., is professor emeritus in cancer biology at Stanford University and pioneered the radiation treatment of cancer with the linear accelerator.

Hyperthermia was pioneered by Ciro Servadio, Ph.D., and Zvi Leib, M.D., of the Beilinson Medical Centre, Petah Tiqva, Israel.

These pioneers should be contacted if you need some expert opinions on various facets regarding the diagnosis and treatment of prostate cancer.

QUESTION: Until my physician told me I had prostate cancer, I felt fine. However, I still do not have any symptoms. What are the symptoms of prostate cancer?

ANSWER: That is one of the problems associated with prostate cancer. During the early stages of the disease, there may be no symptoms. However, after the disease has progressed and you really begin to experience symptoms, you may have missed an opportunity to be cured of the disease because it may have spread to other parts of the body. This is why it is important for all men fifty years of age and older to get an annual physical examination that includes a digital rectal examination and PSA blood test. Among African-American men, I recommend that this physical examination begin at forty. The following may be symptoms associated with prostate cancer; however, they may also be related to other diseases associated with the bladder and urinary tract. You should consult your physician at once if you have any of these symptoms.

- frequent urination
- urgent need to urinate
- waking several times at night to urinate
- incomplete emptying of urine
- hesitation before urination begins
- dribbling after urinating
- decreased size and force of urination
- blood in urine
- painful urination

Finally, a symptom that may mean you have prostate cancer that has spread to your pelvis, ribs, or spine is severe bone or back pain.

QUESTION: My doctor has prescribed combination hormonal therapy, consisting of luprolide and flutamide; however, after two months of treatment with this therapy, I have suffered severe diarrhea. Do you have any suggestions to relieve me of this side effect?

ANSWER: Your diarrhea is probably due to the lactose that is in flutamide. Ask your doctor about the following:

- Avoiding dairy products.

- Using Metamucil.

- Adding Proscar to luprolide and flutamide.

- Discontinuing flutamide.

- Investigating cytadren, cyproterone, and casodex.

- Requesting your doctor to prescribe and order nilutamide for you by calling (418) 656-4141, extension 7818. (Although not approved by the FDA, this drug has been found to be an acceptable substitute for flutamide in Canada.)

QUESTION: I am currently on luprolide and flutamide to treat my prostate cancer. However, throughout the day, I have incidents of hot flashes followed by perspiration. What can I do to cure this condition?

ANSWER: In a study conducted by Drs. Raul Parra and John Gregory from the Division of Urology of the Department of Surgery, St. Louis University Medical Center, and cited in the *Journal of Urology* (vol. 143), 7 patients were treated with clonidine. In 42 percent of the patients, the hot flashes stopped and in the remaining 58 percent, the number and incidence of attacks were greatly reduced. In addition, no side effects were encountered. Approximately 34 percent of men treated with luprolide or a similar drug will experience hot flashes, and in about 30 percent of these patients, the hot flashes will be severe enough to warrant treatment. This equates to about 10 percent of patients on luprolide.

Hot flashes are usually shortlived, often last for a few minutes, and can be precipitated by environmental changes or other stressors. Clonidine is administered by placing a patch on your skin for a 7-day period. The recommended dosage is 0.1 mg. You should consider depo-provera or megace.

QUESTION: What causes treatment refraction?

ANSWER: Refraction is when a prostate cancer victim's treatment is no longer controlled by the current therapy. Sometimes the term progression is used to denote a similar situation in which the prostate cancer continues to grow after a previous response to treatment. If flutamide is the previous treatment, it may be due to the body metabolizing the medication, thereby altering its therapeutic value, or, the body may have developed a tolerance to the medication. The body may harbor prostate cancer cells that may not be sensitive to hormones. Once the ratio of hormone-sensitive cells are less than hormone-insensitive cells, treatment refraction begins. If this is the case, the focus should be on getting appropriate therapy to treat the hyposensitive, hypersensitive, or insensitive prostate cancer cells. This is not to say that combination hormonal therapy should be discontinued, because hormone-sensitive cells will always be in the body until they are totally destroyed.

QUESTION: I have recently received surgery for my prostate cancer. My doctor indicated that I have been cured of the disease. Should I continue participating in my prostate cancer support group?

ANSWER: I personally would if I were you. Although your physician might have pronounced you cured of prostate cancer, there have been countless number of "cured" prostate cancer patients who have had a recurrence of the disease. If you do not want to continue participating in your support group, I would advise you to keep track of your PSA level either on a three- or six-month basis. After a radical prostatectomy, your PSA level should be close to zero ng/ml. As indicated elsewhere in this book, a steady rise of your PSA level over a period of time may indicate a recurrence of prostate cancer.

QUESTION: I have been told by my oncologist that most physicians do not properly stage their prostate cancer patients and this has been verified to some extent by some studies.

ANSWER: An important source I used to conduct my research is a text used by physicians and medical students entitled *Cancer of the Prostate*, by Sakti Das (New York: Marcel Dekker, 1993). This book maintains that the ideal staging of prostate cancer should consist of an accurate assessment of any marginal prostate cancer and an assessment of the lymph nodes. Once the prostate gland and seminal vesicles have been removed, thin slices of the entire prostate gland should be assessed to determine if the disease has spread to other organs and bones.

QUESTION: What is (are) the main reason(s) why researchers cannot find a cure for prostate cancer?

ANSWER: There are essentially three reasons:

1) The cause of prostate cancer is unknown.

2) Some prostate cancer cells are microscopic in nature and researchers have not found an effective method to detect and destroy them; and

3) Some prostate cancer cells are dependent on androgens for growth, and can be combatted by eliminating the source of androgen, while other prostate cancer cells are not dependent on androgens to grow. It is this group of cells for which researchers have not found an effective method to eliminate their deadly result on the human body. Although the answer to this question is simple and direct, the task is horrendous.

QUESTION: What is the cost of a radical prostatectomy and external beam radiation?

ANSWER: The cost varies across geographic areas and among hospitals. However, both treatments cost from $20,000 to $30,000. I might add, however, that the cost for nontraditional treatments for prostate cancer may be as much as 30 to 50 percent less than that of traditional treatments. The cost for the BPH may range from $5,000 to $8,000.

QUESTION: My friend said that he no longer has prostate cancer because of a certain diet he has been on. Could this be true?

ANSWER: Your friend may have had "spontaneous regression." This is a phenomenon in which a person's disease disappears without any treatment. PAACT maintains that the chance of this happening is calculated to be about 1 in 80,000 cases. However, I have not heard of any patients who have been cured of prostate cancer as a result of this phenomenon.

QUESTION: I understand that the doctor can only feel certain parts of the prostate gland, and that this is a significant reason why an annual physical examination should also include a PSA blood test. Is there any truth to this?

ANSWER: Yes. In fact, the prostate gland is divided into three section or zones: 1) the outer zone, which comprises about 65 percent of the prostate; 2) the inner zone, which comprises about 25 percent of the prostate; and 3) the transition zone, which comprises about 5 to 10 percent of the prostate of young adults. The rear posterior portion of the prostate gland can be felt through the rectum by a digital rectal examination. However, the anterior portion of the gland cannot be examined in this manner.

The prostate gland is divided into zones for two important reasons. The first is that the outer and inner zones can be visualized through an ultrasound machine and is thereby a convenient system for establishing a base point for study. The second is that the disease may be biologically different in each of the zones; that is, you may have a well-differentiated tumor in one zone and a moderately differentiated tumor in another zone.

QUESTION: Is three-dimensional radiation therapy an improvement over external beam radiation?

ANSWER: There is no such thing as three-dimensional radiation therapy. I think the best person to respond to this query is George Varsos, M.D., my radiation oncologist. He maintains:

The three-dimensional radiation therapy is merely a software program to aid in treatment planning. It is not to be thought of in contradistinction to external beam therapy because it is a form of external beam therapy using exactly the same linear accelerator. My own editorial comment about the marketing of three-dimensional treatment planning software programs is that the marketers are trying to sell it as something entirely new, which it is not. I have worked with three-dimensional planning programs at Memorial-Sloan Kettering Cancer Center, and put the isodose plans back-to-back against conventional external beam four-field plans, and saw no advantage. The people that market the software and get money for investigating this technique are the main ones who promote it as an entirely different treatment mode. I designed my treatment ports utilizing a treatment planning CT scan at Long Island Jewish Medical Center, or the way that I use the treatment planning MR scan process of transferral of the prostate image onto the isodose computer plan. I personally find the three-dimensional software unnecessary using my technique.

QUESTION: How should I monitor my physical condition after treatment to be alert to a recurrence of prostate cancer?

ANSWER: During the first year of post-treatment, you should visit your physician's office for a digital rectal examination, a urine analysis, and a PSA blood test every three months. You should request these tests at least every six months during the second, third, fourth, and fifth years of post-treatment, and yearly thereafter. In addition, you should also get a transrectal examination and bone scan annually.

Once you begin to do your research, read, and interact with other patients and physicians, you may need answers to other questions. The bibliography of this book may assist you. You should contact PAACT and US TOO, as well.

CHAPTER NINE

What You and Your Partner May Want to Know About the Impact of Prostate Cancer

W hen my wife participated in a group of about 18 other wives who were attending a prostate cancer support group of the Memorial Sloan-Kettering Cancer Center, three very distinct problems or concerns frequently came up among them. These were: how do you deal with a husband who is "incontinenting all over the place?"; what should be done regarding the financial affairs of the household?; and what options are available if the husband is impotent as a result of treatment. These women were frank and expressed a great deal of concern, because it appears that little attention has been given to these matters by the "professionals" and literature. It is not that they were feeling sorry for themselves. My wife said she sensed the entire group felt that life must go on after the consequences of various treatments for prostate cancer and that they, the wives, must be strong and lead the way for their husbands to have a complete recovery after treatment.

In this chapter, I will address each of these concerns, because although I was the cancer victim, my loved ones were affected, too. Because daily living must continue even as you fight the disease, the latter part of the chapter deals with ways to keep healthy, including trying recipes from the National Cancer Institute. I will begin by explaining the side effects of each treatment mentioned in this book. I have also included a section about important business matters you and your spouse should take care of.

COMPLICATIONS WITH COMBINATION HORMONAL THERAPY

If you are receiving combination hormonal therapy to treat your prostate cancer condition, you can expect to be impotent, experience some side effects, and that your sexual drive will wane for the duration of the treatment. To accommodate this condition, several men in my prostate cancer group opted for penile implants. In one case, the injection procedure did not work. All cases reported that their orgasm was different than usual, but was satisfying. In another case, my colleague reported that he suffered pain for two months. In all cases, the wives or companions were elated with the penile implant. I will describe the penile implant procedure later in this chapter.

Combination hormonal therapy will only affect your sexual activities as long as you are undergoing this treatment. Once you stop this treatment, your normal sexual life will be restored. One of my colleagues reported that when he was complaining about the side effects of radiation with Ney, he said, "Well, you can either die with a hard on or live a long and happy life impotent." I guess that sums up what decision has to be made if combination hormonal therapy is your choice; however, you do have another choice. Consider other methods to deal with impotence as described elsewhere in this chapter.

COMPLICATIONS WITH EXTERNAL BEAM RADIATION

If your choice of treatment is external beam radiation and you enjoy a "good" erection prior to treatment, the probability of an "adequate" erection after radiation is quite high. However, you should be mindful that about 50 percent of men who undergo external beam radiation in prostate cancer are impotent afterward. Therefore, unless you and your partner are not sexually active, you should seriously consider other methods to gain an erection and restore your sexual activities.

COMPLICATIONS WITH RADICAL PROSTATECTOMY

If your choice of treatment is radical prostatectomy and your doctor has been trained in nerve-sparing surgery, your sexual life should be regained six to twelve months after the operation. However, if your erection was "weak" prior to the operation, you may lose what "weakness" you had prior to the operation. In cases in which the cancer has spread beyond the prostate, the doctor may find it necessary to avoid the nerve-sparing technique, in order to rid you of any residue of prostate cancer.

When the radical prostatectomy is your choice of treatment, the seminal vesicles, which provide a portion of the sperm, are also extracted along with the prostate gland. If your partner is still of childbearing age and desires to bear children, it is best for you to store sperm in a sperm bank prior to undergoing radical prostatectomy.

However, you and your partner can do the following if you have failed to store sperm in the sperm bank:
1. You and your partner can either have intercourse or mutually masturbate.
2. Immediately after ejaculation, you should urinate into a container.
3. Take the container to a laboratory and have the sperm removed by filtration.
4. Request a doctor to use the sperm to artificially inseminate your wife with the recovered sperm.

Sperm can also be recovered from the bladder through a catheter. This method will have no harmful effects on the sperm. However, because prostate cancer tends to affect most men in their sixties and seventies, fertility is not usually a serious concern.

Another side effect of radical prostatectomy is retrograde ejaculation. If you experience retrograde ejaculation, it is because your sphincter muscle, which is also involved in incontinence, no longer functions properly during intercourse. When the sphincter muscle functions normally, it tightens and closes the passageway through which urine travels to the bladder as semen travels down through the seminal vesicles. When the sphincter is damaged through an operation, the semen follows the line of least resistance and instead of traveling though the penis, travels through the bladder. You can experience normal orgasm, though it is different. Quite often, the only time you may be aware of it is when you see slightly cloudy urine in the toilet bowl when you urinate after intercourse. Some women have been known to complain because they consider it to be dry intercourse.

WHAT YOU CAN DO IF YOU ARE IMPOTENT AS A RESULT OF PROSTATE CANCER

Sometimes men who have undergone radical prostatectomy and external beam radiation are impotent after treatment. If the treatment was combination hormonal therapy, most, if not all men are impotent as long as they are under this specific treatment. Probably because of the disease, as well as the age factor, they may lose interest in all sexual activities.

You will have to do two main things to restore your sexual life together: Revert to an alternative to get an erection and let your partner induce you to perform sexually using a variety of approaches. It is unfair for a husband whose sexual performance has waned because of the aftereffects of treatment to deny his wife sex.

What can be done if you cannot get a "hard" erection after treatment for prostate cancer? Several alternatives are described below.

Get a Penile Implant

This is an invasive technique whereby a penile implant or prothesis is surgically implanted within the penis resulting in an erection sufficiently rigid to engage in sexual intercourse. The operation takes from thirty minutes to two hours. There are four types of implants:

1. The semirigid, which is the simplest of the implants because it can be placed in your penis under local anesthetic and is always ready for use;

2. The malleable, which is made of rods that can be bent and unbent. When you are ready to have sex, all you have to do is unbend the rods. When completed, just bend them back down, allowing your penis to resume a normal position;

3. The self-contained inflatable, which is a more complicated implanted prosthesis that contains a liquid that you pump into two inflatable cylinders in your penis when you have the desire to have sex. After sex, you press a release valve and bend the penis in an effort to get the liquid back into its reservoir; and

4. The fully inflatable, which is the most complicated of all the prostheses. It will allow you to attain a full erection, but also allows it to remain at rest at other times. Its complication rests in its inflatable cylinders. The reservoir for storing the fluid must be inserted in the pelvic region just above the penis. The pump release is located in the scrotum.

Although penile implants can be effective in helping you regain your sexuality, their safety has recently come into question. *Newsday* (November 2, 1993, "Concerns Grow Over the Safety of Implant for Male Impotence," p. 63) reported that:

> the U.S. Food and Drug Administration in April announced that manufacturers of inflatable penile implants—the most popular type—would be required to submit scientific evidence of safety and effectiveness. And soon, the agency will require implant patients to

read and sign an informational letter stating the risks involved, including possible immune system reaction...Inflatable penile implants, which have been around since the early 1970s, are among the first to be scrutinized because they are made of silicone and have generated a high number of consumer complaints— 6,500 since 1984. Moreover, recent studies show that the devices fail and over time may require additional surgery in about one-third of the cases.

Some men in both of my prostate cancer support groups have opted for penile implants. While most have had no complaints, two did indicate that initially they had an infection that lasted two to three months. However, afterward they had no problems. They also indicated that their wives were very satisfied with the implants. Therefore, before you opt for a penile implant, you should thoroughly research the risks.

Inject Medication

A procedure that is getting considerable attention throughout the United States is injection treatment whereby you can inject a medication into your penis each time you want to have intercourse. A medication used for this purpose is papaverine, which is being replaced by prostaglandin E. This allows the erection to subside in less time. The injections are not as bad as they sound. They are painless and very simple to perform. The drawbacks with the injection are that it may not work for every man and it must be spaced twenty-four hours apart. If the erection lasts more than four hours, see a doctor immediately to relieve your penis of some of the blood and to get an antidote. One man was reported as having had an erection for nearly two days and subsequently died.

Use a Suction Pump

With a suction pump, the pump fits over the penis and draws blood into it, creating an erection. An elastic ring is then placed at the base of the penis to contain the blood. This is done each time you want an erection. This erection can last from twenty to thirty minutes. One drawback with this procedure is that it should not be used for more than thirty minutes to prevent damage to the penis.

Consider Penile Bypass

If you are experiencing impotence because of poor blood vessels to the penis, you should consider a surgical procedure to connect one abdominal artery to one or both of the main arteries leading into the penis. The drawbacks with this procedure involve the cost, which is $10,000 to $15,000.

Use Potency Cream

The erectile dysfunction clinic at the New York Hospital of Cornell Medical Center is presently experimenting with a cream that is squeezed into the penis. When all of the cream has gone into the penis, either the husband or wife rubs the penis with the hand until there is an erection. The side effects of this have not yet been determined.

Because the nontraditional treatments for prostate cancer are still in the investigative stages, it is difficult to foresee the complications. Some of the side effects of nontraditional treatments may be identical to traditional treatments, and others may pose little or no complications regarding a patient's sexual life. At any rate, any one of the techniques explained above should be a viable alternative for restoring your sexual life to some extent after a treatment for prostate cancer.

WHAT YOU CAN DO WHEN YOU HAVE A PROBLEM WITH INCONTINENCE

When you undergo radical prostatectomy, you may become incontinent. There are two conditions that may or may not happen to you, but you should know why these occur. The prostate gland is located below the bladder and surrounds the urethra. The urethra is the tube that carries the flow of urine from the bladder and out through the penis. The prostate gland produces a clear fluid that mixes with your sperm prior to ejaculation to produce semen. Although the removal of your prostate gland will not impair your sex drive; it does mean that you will not be able to produce children.

During radical prostatectomy, the urologist will remove the entire prostate gland as well as the seminal vesicles. In addition, he or she will remove part of the urethra that passes through the prostate. The nerves that control the bladder and erections are microscopic in nature and are situated near the prostate gland. Often, if the prostate cancer has spread, the urologist will cut the nerves and sphincter muscle, the structure that enables you to hold your urine in the bladder. In so doing, you may experience permanent loss of bladder control and/or erection difficulty.

One way by which you can deal with bladder problems is to use diapers as a temporary convenience, followed by an AMS sphincter 800 urinary prosthesis, if you are an appropriate candidate. The prosthesis is implanted under your skin. Thousands of men throughout the world are experiencing normal daily voiding activities today using implanted artificial sphincters. The concept behind the artificial sphincter is rather simple. A cuff is implanted around the urethra. It remains closed and keeps the urine in the bladder until you have a desire to urinate. You open the cuff by squeezing a bulb that has been implanted in the scrotum. When the cuff is pumped open, urine flows out of the bladder. The cuff automatically closes within several minutes, keeping the urine in the bladder. But remember, you must be an acceptable candidate for this device.

Wives must be patient with their husbands after surgery and radiation treatment. Even if there is not permanent damage to their bladder or nerves, there may be occasions when they will be incontinent. It is bad enough on the male ego for him to be performing his voiding chores as if he were an infant. An insensitive wife who complains only adds to her husband's stress. A sensitive wife is one who talks less, looks more, and comes up with procedures and ways to help her husband deal with incontinence problems.

If you become incontinent after prostate cancer treatment, there are several things both you and your wife can do to deal with this situation, as described below.

Control Your Diet

Poor diet can lead to incontinence. Too much food and no exercise can lead to obesity, which puts pressure on the bladder. Quite often, a small decrease in weight can be a miracle to incontinence. Constipation can also lead to incontinence. Excellent foods that may help include most fruits, leafy vegetables, whole grain bread, bran cereals, beans, and lentils. Be certain to avoid diuretic foods such as coffee, tea, soft drinks containing caffeine, and alcohol, because they promote incontinence.

Increase Fluid Intake

Make certain you drink lots of water. Schedule your intake of water to your best advantage during the day and do not drink water and other fluids beyond your needs. Two or three quarts of water is sufficient. It is a good idea to limit your water intake to one or two cups after your evening meal.

Some incontinent men tend to limit their intake of fluid, thinking this will help their condition. However, this is a mistake. Too little intake of water will result in dark-colored urine, which will increase your incontinence problem, resulting in constipation. Make certain you void before going to a social event, and to be safe, wear a pad inside your shorts.

Make certain you clean the area of your body that is exposed to the urine. If you are incontinent, cleanse the area with plain soap and water followed by a cream to protect the skin and to avoid odor.

External Collection Devices

An external collection device is made of rubber and resembles a condom. This device is pulled over the penis and held in place by a band around the waist. A tube for drainage is connected to the device and to a collection bag that is secured to your leg by a band. In addition, an external collection device can be used with a penile clamp to control the flow of urine. If this is the choice you and your partner make, be certain you clean yourself frequently and replace parts of the system frequently. If the penile clamp is used, make certain you do not apply too much pressure because it might restrict blood flow through your penis. While some men favor the external collection devices, others do not.

Consider Collagen Implant

If all other attempts to curtail your incontinence have not succeeded, why not try the collagen implant? Collagen implants are made from collagen, which is obtained from cows and is subsequently highly purified for human use. Collagen is a natural protein that when injected into the body of the urethra, reinforces the sphincter muscle by adding bulk, thereby preventing leakage when the bladder muscle has been damaged due to surgery. However, it will be necessary for you to undergo certain tests to determine if the treatment is appropriate and safe for you. These tests will include a physical examination, a medical history, test of urine flow, and a skin test. The skin test is performed to make certain that you are not allergic to the collagen implant. To perform this skin test, your physician will inject a small amount of collagen implant under the skin of your forearm, and is observed for a period of at least four weeks prior to treatment.

The FDA requires all doctors who perform collagen implants to receive specific training before they perform this injection procedure; therefore, do not be hesitant to ask your doctor if he has obtained the proper training. The implant is a rather simple procedure and can be done under local anesthesia. It usually takes 1 to 3 injections and is administered in a 30-minute outpatient procedure. During the clinical trials, 90 percent to 96 percent of the patients showed initial improvement. After a year, about 75 percent of them showed improvement of their condition. When 148 patients were followed up for 2 years, 25 percent to almost 50 percent of them remained dry.

KEGEL EXERCISES

Arnold H. Kegel, M.D., a gynecologist, developed the Kegel exercises to help pregnant women overcome incontinence. Subsequently, the exercises were found to be beneficial for men with prostate cancer. Kegel exercises are performed by tensing and tightening the muscles in the vicinity of the rectum. In the event that you are unaware of this muscle, let me familiarize you with it. This is the muscle you strain when you start or stop urine flow when you are urinating. When exercising this muscle, you should tighten it to a count of five and relax it several times.

What You Can Do When You Have a Problem With Diarrhea

Although I did not experience any diarrhea when I received external beam radiation, a minority of prostate cancer patients will occasionally suffer from radiation effects to the rectum and bladder. Problems with the rectum seem to occur less frequently than with the bladder. Symptoms of the rectum are generally those producing frequency of bowel movement or diarrhea. The following are steps you can take to alleviate diarrhea:

- Drink only clear liquids, such as water, gelatins, or clear broth, which restore fluids in the body depleted with diarrhea. Avoid hot and cold drinks.
- Avoid foods that can give you gas, cause cramps, and irritate your bowels; that is, stay away from cereals high in fiber, raw vegetables, fruits, coffee, and milk products.

- Eat food rich in potassium, such as bananas, potatoes, and apricots. These foods will give you the important minerals necessary for your body to function properly.

- Eat small amounts of food often throughout the day as opposed to large meals less frequently.

- Eat rice, bananas, apple sauce, dry toast, mashed potatoes, and crackers whenever you are stricken with diarrhea.

Healthful Recipes

The following are suggested recipes of the National Cancer Institute for patients that provide the proper nutrients needed during and after treatment for cancer to avoid problems with constipation, diarrhea, and incontinence.

Macaroni and Cheese

1 cup milk
1 tbsp. flour
1-2 tbsp. margarine
1 tsp. minced onion
Salt and pepper to taste

1 tsp. dry mustard (optional)
2 cups elbow macaroni,
    cooked and drained
1 cup shredded cheddar cheese

Measure milk into the pan and blend in flour until no lumps remain. Add margarine, onion, and other seasonings, and cook until sauce thickens. Stir in macaroni and cheese. Bake in greased 1-quart casserole dish, uncovered, at 400 degrees for 15 minutes, or until slightly browned and bubbly. May be frozen before baking. Serves 4.

Cheesy Hamburger Casserole

1 cup macaroni, uncooked
1/2 lb. ground meat
1/2 small onion

3/4 cup tomato sauce or
    chopped tomatoes
1/2 can (10 ounces) cheddar
    cheese soup

Cook macaroni until slightly tender. Drain, set aside. Brown ground meat and onions in small skillet. Add tomatoes and simmer 10 minutes. Oil a 1-quart casserole dish, and spoon in 1.3 ounces of meat mixture. Spread cheese soup over all (may be frozen, unbaked). Cover the casserole tightly and bake at 400 degrees for about 35 minutes. Serves 4.

Cheese-Spinach Pie

1/3 cup chopped onion
1 tbsp. margarine
1/4 lb. sliced cheese
  (Swiss or Muenster)
1 cup cooked, chopped
  spinach, drained

3 large eggs
1/3-1/2 cup of milk
1/2 tsp. salt
Dash pepper

Cook onion in margarine until tender; cool. Lay slices of cheese over pie dough, follow with spinach, then onions. Beat eggs, adding enough milk to make 1 cup. Add seasonings and pour over ingredients in the pie shell. Bake in 400 degree oven about 3 minutes, or until a knife comes out clean. Serve piping hot. (Can be frozen after baking.) Serves 4.

Variation: Substitute cooked, chopped broccoli, green beans, zucchini, or peas for spinach.

Basic Meatloaf or Meatballs

2 tbsp. dry bread or
  cracker crumbs
1 tbsp. water
1/2 lb. ground beef
1 egg

1/4 tsp. minced onion
Salt and pepper to taste
1 tbsp. oil or margarine
2 slices onion

Combine crumbs and water in small mixing bowl. Add meat, minced onion, egg, and seasonings. Mix until well blended. Form into patties, 1-inch meatballs, or a loaf. Brown in oil or margarine in skillet, turning to brown both sides. Add sliced onion, lower heat, cover, and simmer for at least 15 minutes; 30 minutes for meatloaf. You can also bake at 350 degrees.

For meatballs, bake 30 minutes, turning after 15 minutes. For meatloaf, bake 1 hour. Can be frozen raw or cooked. Serves 4.

Sloppy Joes

1/2 lb. ground meat	1/2 cup quick barbecue sauce
1 small onion, diced	1 tbsp. raw oatmeal

Brown meat and onion in skillet. Add barbecue sauce, oatmeal, and enough water to cover meat. Heat to boiling, turn down heat to simmer, cover pan, and cook 15 minutes or until thickened and meat is soft. Serve on buns, toast, or hard rolls. Can be frozen after cooking. Serves 4.

Swedish Meatballs

1 lb. ground round steak	1 egg, slightly beaten
1/2 cup plain bread crumbs	2/3 tsp. salt
1 tbsp. margarine	Dash pepper and allspice

Mix all ingredients except margarine with a fork until well blended. Form into balls, brown in margarine in medium-sized skillet. Remove meatballs from pan. Make a thickened gravy with the drippings. Return meatballs to gravy and simmer, covered, for 1 to 1-1/2 hours. May be frozen raw or cooked. Serves 4.

Chicken Supreme

1 can (10 oz.) cream of mushroom soup	1 cup rice, uncooked
	6 pieces chicken
1/2 cup orange juice	1/4 envelope onion soup mix
1/2 cup water	

Combine first four ingredients and pour into greased 2-quart casserole dish. Lay chicken on top. Sprinkle with dry onion soup mix. Cover casserole, airtight, with heavy aluminum foil. Bake 2 hours without opening foil, at 350 degrees. Can be frozen after baking. Serves 6.

Chicken Skillet Supper

2-3 lbs. frying chicken, cut up	2 sprigs of parsley
1/2 can (10 oz.) vegetable soup	1 basil leaf (optional)
	1 can water

Place chicken, skin side down, in cold skillet. Brown over medium heat, turning to brown inside. Remove from heat (chicken skin can easily be removed at this point if you wish). Pour off all fat remaining in skillet. Replace chicken, pour soup and water over chicken, and add seasonings. Simmer 1 hour in covered skillet, turning pieces once to keep them moist. May be frozen after cooking. Serves 4.

Tomato special: Substitute 1/2 can of cream of tomato for vegetable soup. Add 1 package (10 oz.) of mixed frozen vegetables with the soup and water.

Creamy chicken: Substitute 1/2 can of cream of chicken for vegetable soup, add 1 package (10 oz.) frozen peas and carrots.

Tuna Bake

1 can (7 oz.) water-packed tuna, broken in small pieces	1/4 lb. American or cheddar cheese
1 can (10 oz.) tomato soup	1 lb. box of elbow macaroni, cooked
1 cup milk	

Mix first four ingredients in saucepan and heat until cheese melts. Add macaroni to sauce and mix well. Pour into greased baking dish and bake at 350 degrees for 20 minutes. Serves 8.

Chicken noodle bake: Substitute cream of celery soup for tomato, 1 cup diced chicken for tuna, cooked noodles for elbow macaroni.

Egg noodle bake: Substitute cream of chicken soup for tomato, 3 or more sliced hardboiled eggs for tuna, and cooked noodles for elbow macaroni.

Tuna Broccoli Casserole

2 pkgs. (10 oz.) frozen broccoli, whole or chopped
2 cans (7 oz.) water-packed tuna, broken in small pieces
1 can (10 oz.) cream of mushroom soup diluted with 1/2
    cup milk
1 cup grated cheddar or American cheese
1/2 cup plain bread crumbs
2 tbsp. melted margarine

Cook broccoli according to package directions, drain, and place in shallow 2-quart casserole dish. Add tuna and cover with diluted mushroom soup. Sprinkle with cheese. Add bread crumbs to melted butter and sprinkle over casserole. Bake at 350 degrees for 20 minutes. Serves 5.

Creamy Potato Salad

1/3 cup plain lowfat yogurt
1/3 cup mayonnaise
1/4 tsp. finely minced or
    scraped onion
1 sprig of parsley, finely
    chopped

1/3 cup chopped celery or
    green pepper (optional)
2 potatoes, boiled and diced
2 hard boiled eggs, diced
Salt to taste

Blend yogurt, mayonnaise, onion, parsley, celery, and pepper. Stir in remaining ingredients. Cover and refrigerate for several hours. Serves 4.

Ricotta Potato Salad: Add 1/3 cup ricotta cheese to mayonnaise.

Creole Sauce

1/2 small onion, sliced
1 or 2 frying peppers
(1 bell pepper) cleaned
    and sliced
2 tbsp. oil
2 cups chopped fresh tomatoes,
    or 15-oz. can of tomatoes

1/2 tsp. salt
2 tbsp. sugar
1 tsp. vinegar
1 tbsp. cornstarch
Water

Fry onion and peppers in oil until onion is clear and pepper is spotted with brown. Add tomatoes, salt, sugar, and vinegar. Bring to boiling, turn down to simmer. Cover and cook at least 20 minutes to blend the flavors. Thicken just before serving with cornstarch dissolved in a little water. Use on eggs or meat. Makes 2 cups (1/2 = 1 serving).

Quick Barbecue Sauce

1/2 cup catsup	1/2 tsp. lemon juice
2 tsps. salad style mustard	1 tbsp. brown sugar
1.2 tsp. onion salt	

Mix together in small saucepan. Heat until boiling, stirring as it cooks.

Serving suggestions: Make Sloppy Joes. Use as a barbecue sauce for hot dogs, chicken, or meatballs. (It will easily coat 9 pieces of chicken.) Use as a marinade for chicken or meat: pour over pieces in a deep dish, and refrigerate in marinade, at least 12 hours to tenderize. Makes 1/2 cup.

Sweet and Sour Sauce

1/4 cup vinegar	1/2 tsp. salt
1 cup catsup	1 can (8-oz. size) pineapple
1 tbsp. soy sauce	chunks (optional)
1/2 red or green pepper,	Water
cubed	2 tbsp. cornstarch
1/2 cup honey or brown sugar	
(packed)	

Mix all ingredients except cornstarch in saucepan. Bring to boiling, turn down to simmer. Cover and cook at least 20 minutes to blend the flavors. Thicken just before serving with cornstarch dissolved in a little water. Use on eggs or meat. Makes 2 cups (1/2 cup = 1 serving).

High-Protein Pancakes

1/2 cup milk	2 tsps. of oil
2 tbsp. dry milk	1/2-3/4 cups pancake mix
1 egg (2 for a thinner crepe type)	

Measure milk, dry milk, egg, and oil into blender or bowl. Beat until egg is well blended. Add pancake mix. Stir or blend at low speed until mix is wet but some lumps remain. Cook on hot greased griddle or fry pan, turning when firm to brown the other side. These can be kept warm in a warm oven, or in a covered pan on low heat. Makes seven 4-inch pancakes.

Note: If there is batter left over, it will keep for one day in the refrigerator, or it can be made into pancakes, cooled, and wrapped in foil to be frozen for later use. To reheat, leave in foil and place in 450 degree oven for 15 minutes. If using a toaster oven, unwrap them, brush with margarine, and toast as for light toast.

Low-Lactose Pancakes

1 egg (2 for crepe type)	2 tsps. milk-free margarine, melted
1/2 cup soy formula	
1/2 cup milk-free pancake mix	

Into bowl or blender put egg, soy formula, and melted margarine. Beat to blend. Stir in mix until wet but some lumps remain. Cook on greased or oiled pan (use only milk-free margarine, bacon fat, or shortening) until firm enough to turn over. Brown other side. Keep warm in oven or in covered pan on low heat. If you wish to freeze pancakes, follow directions in recipe for High-Protein Pancakes. Makes six 4-inch pancakes.

Fortified Milk

1 quart milk, homogenized or 1 percent lowfat	1 cup instant nonfat dry milk

Pour liquid milk into deep bowl. Add dry milk and beat slowly with beater until dry milk is dissolved (usually less than 5 minutes). Refrigerate. The flavor improves after several hours. Makes 1 quart.

Banana Milkshake

1 whole ripe banana, slice   Vanilla (few drops)
1 cup milk

Measure into blender and blend at high speed until smooth. Serves 1.

Banana-butterscotch: Add 2 tbsp. of butterscotch sauce with banana.

Strawberry Milkshake

1/2 cup frozen strawberries
1 scoop ice cream
1/2 cup milk

Mix or blend until smooth. Serves 1.

High-Protein Milkshakes

1 cup fortified milk   2 tbsp. of butterscotch,
1 generous scoop   chocolate, or your favorite
  ice cream   fruit syrup or sauce
1/2 tsp. vanilla

Measure all ingredients into blender. Blend at low speed about 10 seconds. Makes 1 serving.

Citrus Fake Shakes

1 frozen citrus fruit juice bar (1-1/2 oz.) or 2 bars (1-3/4 oz.)
  same flavor
1/2 cup chilled Isomil or Neomullsoy
1/4 tsp. vanilla

Remove citrus bar from freezer and allow to thaw slightly (about 5-10 minutes until soft). Break bar into pieces into blender. Add other ingredients and blend at low speed for 10 seconds. Makes 1 serving.

Double citrus: You can increase the use of orange juice without drinking it by adding 1 tbsp. frozen orange juice concentrate and 1 tbsp. sugar to the lemon or orange flavor Fake Shake before blending.

Other Fake Shakes

Butterscotch:
1/2 cup chilled or partially frozen Isomil or Neomullsoy
1/4 tsp. vanilla
2 tbsp. milk-free butterscotch sauce

Blend all at low speed about 10 seconds. Using the partially frozen liquid will produce a much colder, thicker shake. Makes 1 serving.

Chocolate:
Use 2 tbsp. Hershey's chocolate syrup in place of butterscotch. (Commercial chocolate syrups are often made without milk or lactose, but always read the ingredient labels.)

Butterscotch Banana:
Add 1/2 well-ripened, sliced banana to ingredients for butterscotch shake.

Peanut Butter-Honey:
Omit butterscotch sauce. Mix together in a cup: 1/3 cup soy formula or nondairy creamer, 2 tbsp. smooth peanut butter, 1 tbsp. honey, and 1/4 tsp. vanilla. Place partially frozen liquid in blender, then add peanut butter mixture. Blend for about 10 seconds, or until smooth.

Fake Shake Sherbet:
Follow recipe for Peanut Butter-Honey above (you can double or triple recipe easily to save time). Pour shake into small container. Freeze 2 hours or until it begins to harden

around edges. Scrape into bowl and mix thoroughly, until lumps disappear. Return to container and refreeze 2 hours or until firm.

Fake Shake Ice Cream
     Any of the shakes above can be frozen into ice creams, using the same method as for Fake Shake Sherbet.

Fruit Smith

2 tbsp. blackberry or cherry cordial
3/4 cup chilled or partially frozen half-and-half

     Mix or blend until smooth. Serve in a frosted glass, if you like. Serves 1.

Panamanian Smith:
Omit cordial; add tbsp. chocolate syrup and 2 tbsp. rum.

Creme de Menthe Smith:
Omit cordial; add 2 tbsp. creme de menthe and 2 tbsp. vanilla ice cream (omit ice cream for low lactose).

Amaretto Cream

1/2 cup chilled half-and-half2 tbsp. vanilla ice cream
1 tbsp. Amaretto cordial

     Mix until smooth. Serve in stemmed glass. Serves 1.

Butterscotch Brandy Creme:
Omit Amaretto; add 2 tbsp. butterscotch sauce and 1 tbsp. brandy.

Fresh Peach Sauce

1 large peach, peeled and thinly sliced	1/4 cup water
	1 tsp. cornstarch
1-1/2 tbsp. sugar	Dash nutmeg

Combine ingredients in a small pan, stir until cornstarch is dissolved. Cook over medium heat until sauce boils and is thickened. Serves 1.

Milk-Free Butterscotch Sauce

1/3 cup brown sugar,
  packed
2 tsps. cornstarch
1/4 cup nondairy creamer

1/4 cup water
1 tbsp. honey
1 tbsp. milk-free margarine

Mix brown sugar and cornstarch in small saucepan. Slowly add nondairy creamer and water, stirring until cornstarch dissolves. Add honey and margarine. Cook over medium heat, stirring constantly, until sauce is thickened and comes to a boil. Remove from heat. Add vanilla. Cool and store in a covered container in refrigerator. Makes about 1/2 cup.

Milk-free Chocolate: Stir in 1 heaping tbsp. cocoa with cornstarch. If too thick, add a little water after it comes to a boil.

Peanut Butter Snack Spread

1 tbsp. instant dry milk
1 tsp. water
1 tsp. vanilla

1 tbsp. honey
3 heaping tbsp. creamy
  peanut butter

Combine dry milk, water, and vanilla, stirring to moisten. Add honey and peanut butter, stirring slowly until liquid begins to blend with peanut butter. Spread between graham crackers or milk lunch crackers. The spread can also be formed into balls, chilled, and eaten as candy. Keeps well in refrigerator, but is difficult to spread when cold. Makes 1/3 cup.

Molasses taffy flavor: Substitute molasses for honey.

Granola I

1-1/2 cups quick oatmeal
1/2 cup regular wheat germ
1/2 cup coconut
1/2 tsp. salt

1/2 cup chopped nuts
2 tbsp. oil
2/3 cup sweetened
  condensed milk

Measure oatmeal, wheat germ, coconut, salt, and nuts into mixing bowl, stirring to blend. Add oil and mix thoroughly. Pour condensed milk and blend well. Sprinkle a handful of wheat germ on a cookie sheet and gently spread mixture on top. Bake in 325 degree oven, about 25 minutes. Check mix as it bakes—after the first 10 minutes, mix will begin to brown. Stir it on cookie sheet every 10 minutes until it is as brown as you like. Cool on pan; store in covered container in refrigerator.

Granola II: Omit milk. Add 1/2 cup honey. Bake as above.

Chocolate chip: Put hot mixture in bowl. Stir in 1/2 cup of chocolate chips.

Raisin: Stir in 1 cup of raisins after the mixture cools.

Granola Bars

3/4 cup quick oatmeal	1 egg
1/2 cup Granola II	1/4 tsp. vanilla extract
1/2 cup coconut	1 tbsp. honey
1/2 cup brown sugar (packed)	1/4 tsp. salt
1/4 melted margarine	1/4 cup flour

Measure oatmeal, granola, coconut, and brown sugar together in deep bowl. Mix well. Pour melted margarine over all and blend thoroughly. Beat the egg, extract, honey, and salt together. Pour this over dry ingredients, stirring to blend. Add flour, stirring until smoothly mixed. Press mixture onto greased, floured 11 x 17-inch shallow baking pan or cookie sheet. Bake at 325 degrees for 35 minutes. Cool slightly, cut into bars, and remove from the pan while warm. Makes 18 bars.

Apple Brown Betty

4 cups thinly sliced pared apples or 1 can (16 oz.) pie apples, drained	1/2 cup brown sugar, packed
	1/8 tsp. brown sugar
	2 tbsp. margarine
	1/4 cup hot water
2 cups bread cubes or torn bread pieces.	

Grease 1-quart baking dish. Arrange half of apples on bottom of dish. Follow with half of bread, then half of sugar. Repeat layers. Sprinkle cinnamon over top, cut margarine in pieces and lay them on top, finish by pouring hot water over all. Cover and bake at 350 degrees for 30 minutes, uncover, and bake 10 minutes longer. Serve warm or chilled. Serves 4.

Apple Cheese Betty: Spoon 1 cup ricotta cheese over first layer of apples, bread, and sugar. Complete as above.

Apple Raisin Cake

1-3/4 cups coarsely chopped apples, or drained canned pie apples, chopped	1 tsp. baking powder
	1/2 tsp. salt
	1-1/2 cups flour
	1 tsp. cinnamon
3/4 cup brown sugar, packed	1/2 tsp. nutmeg
1/2 cup oil	1/2 cup raisins, plumped
1 egg, beaten	in warm water
1/2 tsp. baking soda	

Measure apples and brown sugar into bowl. Add oil and eggs. Add dry ingredients and mix well. This dough will be stiff. Add raisins and nuts. Stir to blend. Spread in 8-inch square pan. Bake at 350 degrees or until top springs back when touched. May be frozen. Makes 16 pieces.

Individual Cheese Pie

1 tbsp. ricotta cheese	2 tsps. sugar
1 tbsp. applesauce (pureed), peaches, or drained crushed pineapple (store bought)	Sprinkle of cinnamon
	One 3-inch sugar cookie

Blend cheese, fruit, sugar, and cinnamon. Spoon over a sugar cookie, turned upside down so the sugar side is on the bottom next to the cookie sheet or foil. Bake at 350 degrees for 15 minutes (the cookie softens as it absorbs the liquid from the fruit-cheese mixture); for a softer treat, lower the oven to 325 degrees. Serves 1.

Banana-Nut Bread

2 eggs	3/4 cup sugar
3 medium well-ripened	1 tbsp. baking powder
bananas cut into chunks	1/2 tsp. baking soda
1/4 cup of milk	1/2 tsp. salt
1/4 cup of oil	1/4 tsp. nutmeg
1 tsp. vanilla extract	1/2-1 cup chopped walnuts
2 cups all-purpose flour	or pecans, or wheat germ

Blend eggs, bananas, milk, oil, and vanilla at medium speed until smooth, about 15 seconds. Measure rest of ingredients into bowl and stir to mix. Make a well in the center of the dry ingredients and pour in banana mixture. Mix just enough to moisten. Add pan or three small 5 x 3 x 2-inch pans. Bake the bread at 350 degrees, about 1 hour for the large loaf and 35-45 minutes for the smaller ones. Makes 1 large loaf or 3 small loaves (16 slices).

Soft Chocolate Frosting

1/2 cup white sugar	3 heaping tbsp. cornstarch
1/2 cup brown sugar	1 cup milk
3 heaping tbsp. cocoa	3 tbsp. margarine

Mix first four ingredients together in saucepan until well blended. Gradually add milk. Add margarine. Cool over medium heat, stirring constantly until thick and smooth. (You may need to remove from heat occasionally to prevent sticking or lumping.) Ice cake while the frosting is still warm. Ices two 9-inch layers (serving 6 people). Recipe can easily be cut in half for a single layer cake or cupcakes.

Cowboy Cookies

1 cup soft shortening or
  margarine
3/4 cup brown sugar, packed
3/4 cup granulated sugar
2 eggs
1 tsp. vanilla extract
2 cups flour

1/2 tsp. baking soda
1/2 tsp. salt
1-1/2 cups quick oatmeal
1/2 cup coarsely chopped
  nuts or wheat germ
6 oz. chocolate chips
1 cup raisins

Cream shortening, add sugars, and beat well. Add the eggs and vanilla and stir to blend well. Add the dry ingredients at one time. Mix to blend thoroughly. Last, stir in oatmeal, nuts, chocolate chips, and raisins. Mix well. Drop by spoonfuls on cookie sheet and bake for 13-15 minutes in 350 degree oven. This dough freezes well and can be sliced later to make fresh cookies. Makes 4-dozen large cookies.

Peanut Butter Bars

1/4 cup margarine
1/4 cup smooth peanut butter
1-1/3 cups brown sugar,
packed
2 eggs

1-1/2 cups flour
1-1/2 tsps. baking powder
1/2 cup chocolate chips
1/2 cup finely chopped nuts
  (optional)

Cream margarine and peanut butter. Add brown sugar and mix well. Add both eggs and mix until well blended. Stir in dry ingredients until blended, then chocolate chips and nuts. Spread batter in greased and floured 9-inch sauce pans. Bake at 350 degrees for 30-35 minutes. Cool in pan. Cut when cooled into 36 bars.

Fluffy Fruit Gelatin

1 cup cooked or canned peaches with syrup
1 package red gelatin (3 oz.)
1 cup boiling water

Blend fruit with syrup at high speed until smooth. Pour pureed fruit back into measuring cup and add enough syrup or water to make one cup. Dissolve gelatin in boiling water, pour into a bowl (deep enough to whip gelatin later). Stir in fruit puree. Cool. Refrigerate gelatin mixture until it piles softly, but is not firm. With cold beaters, whip the gelatin until foamy and doubled in volume. Refrigerate until firm. Serves 6.

Other fruits: Use pears, applesauce, or apricots in place of peaches.

Fluffy Fruit Cream: Fold in 1 cup of whipped cream or nondairy whipped topping after whipping the gelatin. Refrigerate until firm.

Rice Pudding

1 tbsp. cornstarch	1 cup milk
1-1/2 tbsp. granulated sugar	1/2 cup well-cooked rice
1 beaten egg	1/2 tsp. vanilla

Blend first three ingredients in saucepan until smooth. Add milk slowly, stirring to mix well. Add rice. Cook over medium heat, stirring constantly until mixture is thickened and comes to a boil. Remove from heat, add vanilla, and cool. Sprinkle with cinnamon and nutmeg if desired. Many prefer rice pudding warm. Try it for a new taste treat. Makes 3 servings.

Milk-free Double Chocolate Pudding

2 squares baking chocolate (1 oz. each)	1/2 cup granulated sugar
1 tbsp. cornstarch	1 cup nondairy creamer or soy formula
1 tsp. vanilla	

Melt chocolate in small pan or on foil. Measure cornstarch and sugar into saucepan. Add part of the creamer and stir until cornstarch dissolves. Add the remainder of the creamer. Cook over medium heat until warm. Stir in chocolate until mixture is thick and comes to a boil. Remove from heat. Blend in vanilla, and cool. Makes 2 servings.

Milk-free Vanilla Pudding

1/4 cup sugar   1 egg, beaten
2 tbsp. cornstarch   1 tsp. vanilla
2 cups Isomil or Neomullsoy

Measure sugar and cornstarch into saucepan. Add a little of the soy formula. Stir to dissolve cornstarch, then pour in the rest of the liquid. Add beaten egg. Cook over medium heat until it comes to a boil and is thickened. Add vanilla and cool. Makes 4 servings.

Maple pudding: Omit vanilla and add 1/2 tsp. maple flavoring.

Maple-Nut pudding: Add 1/4 to 1/2 cup chopped walnuts or pecans to cooled pudding. (Not permitted on soft diet).

Coconut pudding: Add 1/2 cup coconut. Read the ingredient listing on coconut to be sure it has no lactose added. (Not permitted on soft diet).

Super Frozen Delight

1 pkg. instant pudding   2 cups of chilled Isomil or
  (chocolate, vanilla,   Neomullsoy
  butterscotch, or lemon)   2 cups nondairy whipped
                                  topping

Read the label of pudding mix to see that no milk or other milk product has been included. Prepare pudding as directed, substituting Isomil or Neomullsoy for milk. Gently fold in whipped topping. Pour into freezer container, cover, and freeze until firm, about 3 hours. Makes 2 quarts (8 servings).

Nut Delight:Fold in 1 cup of your favorite chopped nuts with the whipped topping. (Not permitted on soft diet.)

IMPORTANT BUSINESS MATTERS YOU
AND YOUR PARTNER SHOULD DISCUSS

While it is difficult to consider the possibility of death from prostate cancer, it is fair to your family to put your affairs in order. In view of the 35,000 men who will die of prostate cancer annually and because you may have to deal with certain problems, in this section, I will suggest some specific things, mostly financial, that you and your partner should consider doing if you have prostate cancer.

1. Collect all life insurance policies and make certain they are paid up to date. Further, identify to your partner all accounts you have with life insurance coverage. If you are not certain if you have life insurance or a particular account, contact the company to find out.

2. Take your name off your safe deposit box to prevent the government from seizing it.

3. Take out a disability insurance policy with the American Association of Retired Persons (AARP) so if you do go into the hospital, your partner can collect a weekly sum from the insurance company.

4. Try to get some burial insurance to reduce costs for burial.

5. Make certain all your state and federal tax returns have been filed and ascertain if any taxes are due and for what period. Pay them.

6. Keep your jewelry and other valuables in a safe place where your partner can get them.

7. Look to determine if there are any pictures of you with other members of the family. If you have none, get one done as soon as possible.

8. Locate a copy of your discharge papers in the event you want to get buried at a military base.

9. Make out a living will, prepare a health care proxy, and sign over to your partner the power of attorney.

10. Meet with your partner to identify all of your checking accounts and to surrender all bank books to her care.

11. Give your partner the mortgage and deeds of any real estate property you own and store them in a secure place.
12. Update your will if deemed necessary.
13. Identify certain mementos for certain members of the family.
14. List on paper anything you desire done after your death.
15. Record a videotape to deliver an important message to your immediate family.
16. List all stocks and bonds, indicating name, location, and date of purchase.
17. Meet with the family to discuss any upcoming financial dealings.
18. Declare in writing to your partner all past and future financial losses that are or can be reported on your federal and state tax returns.
19. Complete a balance sheet on your assets and liabilities. You may need an accountant to help with this item.
20. Inform your partner as to the location of all charge cards and keep those not often used in a safe place.

Important Documents

If you are undergoing any operation, or if you have a Stage D1, D2, or D3 disease, you should prepare a health care proxy and store it in a secured location. Some states have a health care proxy law that allows you to appoint someone you trust, like a family member or close friend, to decide about your treatment if you lose the ability to decide for yourself. You can do this by using a health care proxy form. Your hospital may have to appoint your health care agent. In many instances, it will be your wife. This law gives you the power to make sure that health care professionals follow your wishes. Hospitals, doctors, and other health care providers must follow your agent's decisions as if they were your own. You can give the person you select as little or as much authority as you want. You can also allow your agent to decide about all health care concerns or only certain treatments. You may also give your agent instruction that he or she has to follow.

What is the difference between health care proxy and a living will? A living will is a document that provides specific instructions about health care treatment. It is generally used to declare wishes and to indicate that you would refuse life-sustaining treatment under certain circumstances. In contrast, the health care proxy allows you to choose someone you trust to make treatment decisions on your behalf. Unlike a living will, a health care proxy does not require you to know in advance all the decisions that may arise. Instead, your health care agent can interpret your wishes as medical circumstances change and can make decisions you could not have known would have to be made. The health care proxy is just as useful for decisions to receive treatment as it is for decisions to stop treatment. If you complete a health care proxy form but also have a living will, the living will provides instructions for your health care agent, and will guide his or her decisions. If you want a living will, get an attorney to produce one for you, or purchase a do-it-yourself kit.

A health care proxy is important because if you become too sick to make health care decisions, someone else must decide for you. Health care professionals often look to family members for guidance. But family members are not allowed to decide to stop treatment, even when they believe that is what you would choose or what is best for you under the circumstances. Appointing an agent lets you control your medical treatment by:

- Allowing your agent to stop treatment when he or she decides that is what you would want or what is best for you under the circumstances.

- Choosing one family member to decide about treatment because you think that person would make the best decisions or because you want to avoid conflict or confusion about who should decide.

- Choosing someone outside your family to decide about treatment because no one in the family is available or because you prefer that someone other than a family member decides about your health care.

Your health care agent would begin to make treatment decisions after doctors decide that you are not able to make them yourself. As long as you are able to make treatment decisions, you will have the right to do so. You can appoint your health care agent without an attorney. All you need is two adult witnesses.

You can write instructions on the proxy form. Your agent must follow oral and written instructions, as well as your moral and religious beliefs. If your agent does not know your wishes or beliefs, your agent is legally required to act in your best interests.

Because you might change your mind about your health care decision, it is easy to cancel the proxy, change the person you have chosen as your health care agent, or change any treatment instruction you have written on his health care proxy form. Just fill out a new form. In addition, you can require that the health care proxy expire on a specified date or if certain events occur. Otherwise, the health care proxy will be valid indefinitely. If you choose your spouse as your health care agent and you get divorced or legally separated, the appointment is automatically cancelled.

You will also want to prepare a last will and testament. If you and your partner already have a will, review it together to update it. You may wish to bequeath some money to PAACT or to some other nonprofit organization that specializes in prostate cancer. If, on the other hand, you and your partner do not have a will, either go directly to your lawyer and make one out or get a do-it-yourself kit and make one out jointly.

Sometimes a prostate cancer patient may have a strong desire to leave personal instructions for his wife to carry out pertaining to a number of other things that are not cited in the last will and testament. You can prepare a "do not open until my death" document. These instructions may be any of the following:

- Burial instructions

- Self-prepared eulogy
- Special love messages to each of the children and your wife
- Press release
- Any secrets you may wish to divulge to the family
- Instructions for each child
- Any other matters

Finally, just in case it may be needed, you should give your partner power of attorney. Most stationery stores have pre-printed power of attorney documents. All you have to do is purchase one, fill out the appropriate blanks, and get it notarized.

As you travel the journey to either curing your disease or lengthening your life, you and your partner must form a partnership to lessen the impact of the prostate cancer on yourselves and others. You must recognize that each treatment carries with it some side effects that the two of you must embrace and deal with in order to make both of your lives as normal as possible. These side effects may affect your sexual lives and may involve incontinence. The impact will certainly affect you and your partner's financial affairs. However, if you use the contents of this chapter as a guideline, both of you will get through any ordeal with strength and determination.

CHAPTER TEN

What You Should Do if You Have a Recurrence of Prostate Cancer

Once when I was attending my prostate cancer support group in New York City, I was somewhat astounded when many of my colleagues related their innermost thoughts regarding the recurrence of prostate cancer and how much (or how little) time they had to live. That night still lingers with me because it enabled me to think about my own mental set. True, I have given some thought to dying, but I can honestly say, it did not stay with me for any length of time. As I ponder why, there are probably several reasons for my healthy attitude as it relates to prostate cancer and death:

1. I have developed a contingency plan as a second chance to battle prostate cancer.
2. I do not linger in the past or future, but practice the theme of "be here now."
3. I am living each day as though it may be my last.
4. I really believe that this life is only a series of lives that the soul experiences, and this experience is coming to an end.
5. Death is a treasure to behold so that I will once again be with God.

These platforms work for me, although they may not work for you. Each person must navigate his own life with or without the help of others to prevent his thoughts about the future from debilitating him now.

Regardless of your treatment for prostate cancer and the stage of your disease, there is always the possibility that your disease can recur. In this chapter, I will discuss some steps that all prostate cancer victims should take if their disease should recur.

HOW DO YOU KNOW IF YOUR DISEASE HAS RECURRED?

There are a number of methods your doctor can use to determine if your prostate cancer has recurred. These include:

1. He or she can give you a digital rectal examination and feel for any nodules, stiffness, enlargement, or hardness of the prostate gland. Although this method may not work for everyone, some recurrences may be detected in some men.

2. As indicated in Chapter One, once you have been treated for prostate cancer and your PSA level has increased .75 ng/ml or less, then your disease may have recurred. However, some doctors will instead look for a rise in the trend of the PSA level to more accurately diagnose a recurrence of the disease.

3. A positive biopsy may signal that your disease has recurred; however, it is possible that your cancer cells are not active. As a result, you may be an appropriate candidate for watchful waiting.

Even though a biopsy may have indicated that you have "positive" prostate cancer cells, a study by Bagshaw maintained that when prostate cancer was confined to the gland, there was no further progression of cancer in 50 percent of 116 patients. The study further indicated that patients subsequently remained alive and well from 2.2 to 22.7 years with a median follow up of 13.8 years. In those patients for whom doctors could detect recurrent nodules via digital rectal examination, the disease most likely had metastasized, which indicated that the tumor had already spread even before the treatment, although it went undetected. However, it has clearly been shown that the time to regression of disease on the pathology slide in radiation therapy is frequently longer than one year. Many of the patients in the Bagshaw Study may have been biopsied early, and thought to have viable cells in the tumor specimen. If some of these patients were biopsied after 18 months, the results could well have been different. However, we have not been able to discern what is viable.

Three types of recurrence can be identified:
1. Microscopic cancer in the prostate with or without an elevated or rising PSA level.
2. Rising PSA level without clinical or microscopic disease in the prostate, although the diseases may be located in the lymph nodes.
3. A cancerous tumor in which nodules can be felt via the digital rectal examination and a rising PSA.

Figure 10.1
Post-treatment PSA Trend Chart

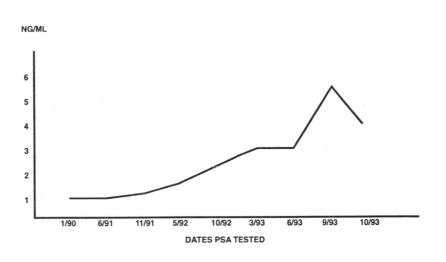

The prostate cancer trend chart illustrated in Figure 10.1 is that of a colleague of mine who is in my prostate cancer support group. His doctor told him he had nothing to worry about because his PSA level is back to 4.0 ng/ml. I told him to get another doctor because there is a high probability that his prostate cancer (after a radical prostatectomy) has recurred. Remember, previously I said that if the PSA level shows a steady rise after treatment, there is a high probability that there is a recurrence of the disease. When a diseased gland has been removed through radical prostatectomy, the PSA level should be nearly zero.

If you have a recurrence of the disease, one of the first things you should consider doing is to request your physician to put you on combination hormonal therapy immediately to slow down the growth, debulk, and downstage your disease. While some doctors only prescribe luprolide as an appropriate therapy, I strongly recommend that you insist that your doctor put you on combination hormonal therapy; that is, luprolide and flutamide. You want to close down the entire system that produces testosterone, not just part of the system. This will enable you to fight your disease on at least two fronts—your testes and your adrenal glands. However, if you have had a bilateral orchiectomy, luprolide will not be necessary.

WHAT CAN YOU DO IF YOUR CANCER HAS RECURRED

Believe it or not, even if you have received radiation to rid yourself of prostate cancer, you may still be a viable candidate for surgery if your disease has recurred. However, before the operation can proceed, you should meet certain conditions, such as those indicated below:

- You should be in excellent health.

- You should have a life expectancy of at least ten years.

- The tumor should not be in a high grade of malignancy because it may be a signal that the disease has spread.

- The seminal vesicles should not be involved with the tumor.

- If the tumor was not operable before radiation, it is probably not operable after the recurrence.

- A rapidly climbing PSA level may indicate that the disease has spread and surgery may not be appropriate.

If your choice of treatment for a recurrence of prostate cancer after external beam radiation is radical prostatectomy, you should consider the following:

- There may be a greater risk of damage to the rectum or bladder; however, these conditions are diminishing with better surgical methods.

- The risk of incontinence may be as high as 50 percent, although this condition can be accommodated with artificial sphincters.

- The doctor should be trained and well experienced with irradiated tumors.

- The survival rate of the subsequent disease rate is approximately 50 percent if the patients have been carefully selected.

Sometimes, in the absence of better alternatives, recurrence of prostate cancer after external beam radiation can be retreated with external beam radiation, according to Dr. Bagshaw. However, this should only be undertaken if you freely understand the increased risk for tissue injury because of reduced tissue tolerance. My urologist maintains that this is very dangerous.

If your choice of retreatment of recurrence of prostate cancer is external beam radiation, cystoscopy and sigmoidoscopy should be performed to determine the condition of your irradiated tissues. At any rate, the total dose of radiation should be reduced. The condition of the rectum and bladder should be reassessed prior to irradiation of tissue. Seed implantation is not an option for those patients who fail radical prostatectomy. The success of seed implantation is based on being able to define clearly a target volume. After the prostate has been removed, there no longer remains a circumscribed area in which the recurrences occur. Be mindful that retreatment of internal beam radiation for recurrence of prostate cancer should only be done at cancer centers that have substantial experience in radiation therapy.

As indicated in Chapter Two, a viable alternative treatment for a recurrence of prostate cancer after external beam radiation could be cryosurgery. Allegheny Hospital in Pittsburgh, Pennsylvania, has treated patients with a recurrence of prostate cancer after radical prostatectomy and external beam radiation. In fact, cryosurgery is my first choice of treatment and seed implantation is my second choice of treatment if there is a recurrence of prostate cancer.

If your first and only treatment of choice was combination hormonal therapy and you have been diagnosed as a Stage A or B patient, depending on your age, you could opt for any of the traditional or nontraditional treatments. If you have been diagnosed as a Stage C patient, depending on the spread of your disease, you should consider either external beam radiation, seed implantation, or cryosurgery. However, if you have been diagnosed as a late Stage D patient and have hormonal refractory disease, PAACT suggest the administration of cytadren plus hydrocortisone supplement as secondary hormonal blockade, monitored by monthly PSA analysis.

Consider Clinical Trials

If you are a Stage D patient and you are getting minimal or no results from current therapies and drugs and your PSA continues to rise, you should look into participating in a clinical trial, of which there are many. They range from studies of ways to prevent, detect, control, and treat cancer to studies of the psychological impact of the disease, as well as ways to improve the patient's quality of life (including pain relief).

Clinical trials are usually divided into four phases. In Phase I, a new treatment is administered to a small number of patients to determine the best way to give the treatment to patients and how much can be given to the patient safely. Although the new treatment may have been given to animals, no one knows for certain how a human patient may react to the same treatment. As a result, Phase I studies are very risky. That is why clinical trials are usually only given to patients whose cancer has metastasized. Some patients who have received Phase I treatments have had positive results.

In Phase I studies, the effects of the new research treatment is determined. Each new phase of a clinical trial is dependent on and builds on the information obtained in the preceding phase. If a new treatment demonstrates some results against cancer in Phase II, it moves to Phase III whereby the new results are compared with the traditional or standard to determine which treatment is more effective. Usually, researchers will use a traditional treatment as the departure point for creating a new and more effective treatment. In Phase IV studies, the new treatment becomes part of the traditional treatment to help patients. For example, a drug found effective in a clinical trial may be used together with other effective treatments, such as radical prostatectomy or radiation, or with another effective drug.

There are numerous ways to determine what clinical trial treatments are available. You can talk with your doctors and obtain opinions from cancer specialists. As mentioned in Chapter Eight, a helpful treatment information system called PDQ is supported by the National Cancer Institute. PDQ will provide your doctor with the most current information on clinical trials being offered in the United States for each type and stage of cancer. However, this system is only available for your doctor.

The Cancer Information Service (CIS) is another source of information. CIS answers cancer-related questions from the public, cancer patients, their families, and health professionals. For additional information, call the toll-free number: 1-800-4-CANCER.

Cancer centers, the National Cancer Institute, universities, community hospitals, and private industries have initiated a number of research studies that may be what you are looking for. If you are interested, you should contact the National Cancer Institute.

PAACT is also a good source for learning of appropriate ongoing or upcoming clinical trials.

A word to the cautious: Clinical trials usually consist of two groups—one who will receive the new treatment, and another that who receive a placebo. As a result, if you participate in a clinical trial, you may not be the one to receive the treatment, therefore consuming valuable time to arrest and treat your disease with a traditional treatment.

What You Should Do to Cope With Bone Pain

It is estimated that 400,000 cancer patients annually in the United States develop bony metastases. About half of these patients experience severe bone pain. I understand the bone pain is similar to that of having a continuous severe toothache. Most treatments for eliminating bone pain have not been effective; as a result, patients usually end up taking some form of a narcotic, becoming addicted to the drug, and sometimes becoming incapacitated. Application of radiotherapy to the area of involved bone may relieve or decrease pain.

There seems to be two effective non-narcotic drugs that relieve prostate cancer patients of bone pain as stated in Chapter Two:

- Metastron, which is distributed by Medi-Physics, Inc.

- Samarium-153-EDTMP, also referred to as CYT-424, which is distributed by the Cytogen Corporation.

Metastron is a radioisotope that relieves bone pain for an average of six months and is administered in a single injection. Once introduced to the body, it goes directly to the site of the cancer cells in the bones. A single dose of Metastron improves pain control in 67 percent to 75 percent of patients. In a multicenter trial, 20 percent of patients with advanced prostate cancer experienced complete relief of bone pain. In addition, repeat injections are also effective. Unlike narcotic remedies,

Metastron does not cause nausea, vomiting, or constipation. The only side effect noted is that in some patients, there is a mild facial flushing, usually occurring when the drug is administered too quickly.

Samarium-153, as well as strontium-89 is a radioisotope that relieves bone pain in 70 to 80 percent of patients within 4 to 7 days and lasts for 4 months. However, Samarium-153 is still in the investigative stages and has not been approved by the FDA.

Join Us Too's High Risers

US TOO has organized a Prostate Cancer Support Group in Chicago called the High Risers. These are men whose disease has recurred. Even if a High Riser chapter is not available at a local hospital in your community, stay in touch with the one in Chicago and arrange to get any of their materials. Better yet, organize your own group of High Risers and support each other. Refer to Chapter Four for more information on US TOO's High Risers.

Execute Your Prostate Cancer Contingency Plan

In Chapter Four, I recommended that if you have been treated for prostate cancer, you should give serious consideration to creating a prostate cancer contingency plan with trigger points. Now is the time to execute that plan. However, before you do, it may be advisable for you to reconsider your contingency treatment based on new research, treatments, and drugs; that is, if you have not already updated your plan. Therefore, before implementation of your plan, speak to your physicians and others about what is new in the treatment of prostate cancer.

Try Integrating Physical Healing With Dietary and Psychological Healings

Although when I first learned I had prostate cancer, fear did sweep over my entire body, after releasing myself of the right side of my brain, which controls my feelings, I began to shift my thoughts to the left side of my brain, which controls the rational side of my thoughts. I realized that I had to learn much about the prostate cancer in order to survive, and if possible, to cure myself of the disease. I also recognized that if I weakened and let negative factors or thoughts invade my being, then the cancer would control me rather than me controlling the disease.

I was very mindful that my thoughts would either weaken or strengthen any medical treatment I might receive from the medical profession. You see, I believe optimal healing for prostate cancer will only result if you integrate your physical healing with dietary and psychological healings. The major portion of this book has dealt with physical healing. This section will give some (although it deserves much more) space to dietary and psychological healings.

There are a number of studies that help to illuminate some causes of prostate cancer as indicated below:

- Seventh Day Adventists who drank two glasses of milk per day had nearly double the risk of prostate cancer as those drinking one glass. And three glasses of milk increased the odds about two-and-one-half times. On the other hand, it was found that Seventh Day Adventist men in California have 55 percent less prostate cancer than other men. Church members tended to avoid meat, poultry, fish, refined foods, alcohol, stimulants, and spices, and consumed whole grains, vegetables, and fresh fruits.

- Researchers at Buffalo-Roswell Park Memorial Institute, who examined the diets of men with prostate cancer and those without, found a relationship to whole milk, but not skim milk. Drinking more than three glasses of whole milk per day increased the cancer risk by two-and-one-half times.

- A British study found that cancer rates dropped by 40 percent in men with the most blood beta carotene, as compared to those with the least.

- Research has found that those with higher levels of folic acid, which is found in green vegetables and lycopere (a type of tomato), are less vulnerable to all kinds of cancer.

- In a controlled study of 45 men, it was found that when they took amino acids in pure form, they experienced a reduction in the major symptoms of prostate enlargement. For example, they relieved or reduced nighttime urination by 15 percent, the need to urinate by 81 percent, and frequency of urination by 73 percent. Amino acids can be obtained from pumpkin seeds, cucumber seeds, watermelon seeds, sesame seeds, soybeans, flax seeds, almonds, and peanuts.

- In a controlled study, it was reported that prostate cancer patients consumed less food high in Vitamin A and beta carotene, such as carrots.

- A report found that counties in the United States with the highest death rates from prostate cancer also had the highest per capita intake of high-fat foods, including beef, milk and dairy products, fats and oils, and pork and eggs.

- A ten-year study of over 120,000 Japanese men over age 40 found less prostate cancer deaths among those who regularly consumed green or yellow vegetables. The study reported that vegetarian men have a lower incidence of prostate cancer than nonvegetarian men.

- More than ten years have elapsed since the National Academy of Sciences concluded, after reviewing research, that: "In summary, the incidence of prostate cancer is correlated with other cancers associated with diet, e.g., breast cancer. There is good evidence that an increased risk of prostate cancer is associated with certain dietary factors, especially the intake of high fat and high protein foods, which usually occur in the diet. There is some evidence that vitamin A or its precursors and vegetarian diets are associated with a lower risk."

Eat a Recommended Diet for Prostate Cancer

In Chapter Nine, I included the National Cancer Institute's recommended general diet for Americans with cancer. In this section, I am going further and recommending that you consider a macrobiotic diet to combat prostate cancer. Michio Kushi, a macrobiotic nutritionist, has written a book entitled, *The Cancer Prevention Diet ... Blueprint for the Relief and Prevention of Disease* (St. Martin's Press, New York: 1983), which makes the following dietary recommendations for prostate cancer. However, my oncologist has stated that there is no hard data supporting this diet as a cure for prostate cancer. He also maintains that it is certainly not for every patient.

Because there is evidence that prostate cancer develops as a result of dietary habits, foods that should be avoided are high in protein and fat, such as all meats, poultry, eggs, cheese, milk and other dairy products. Less fatty animal foods like fish and seafood should also be avoided if at all possible or at least consumed in limited amounts. In addition, sugar, honey, chocolate, carob, and all sugar-treated foods and beverages should be discontinued.

Other foods that have the potential to create mucous, such as refined white bread, pancakes, and cookies, should also be avoided. All stimulants, such as mustard, pepper, curry, mint, peppermint, and other aromatic herbs and spices, all alcoholic beverages, and coffee should be avoided because these enhance tumor growth even though they are not the direct cause of prostate cancer. All foods chemically and artificially treated during production and processing should be avoided. In addition, excessive consumption of salts, salty foods, beverages, and oil (even of the vegetable and unsaturated types) should be avoided.

Be mindful that if fruits and fruit juices are consumed frequently, these can increase the swelling of the prostate gland, although they can neutralize animal protein and fat. However, they should be limited. All vegetables of tropical origin, such as potatoes, tomatoes, eggplant, and subtropical fruits should be avoided.

Consider using shark cartilage to cure or prevent a recurrence of prostate cancer. Although this treatment is still experimental in the United States and other countries, I believe it at least deserves some mention in this book since it is a nontoxic agent that can be purchased in most health food stores. It is believed by several medical doctors and researchers that tumors require a new blood supply to feed their growth, a process called angiogenesis. It appears that sharks for the most part do not get cancer and that their cartilage can be used as an antiangiogenesis agent to reduce the supply of blood to the tumor cells, resulting in starvation and death of tumors.

The anecdotes cited in Dr. I. William Lane's recent book, *Sharks Don't Get Cancer* (Avery Publishing Group, Inc., Garden City Park, New York: 1993), about prevention and cure of cancer with shark cartilage are mixed, meaning that the health of some patients was restored and others received no benefit from it. It is up to each individual reader to decide for himself if shark cartilage should be used to treat advanced stage prostate cancer or to use it as a preventative therapy.

If you intend to use shark cartilage, the recommended dosage is one-half gram multiplied by your weight. For example, my weight is 190 pounds; therefore my recommended daily dosage would be 1/2 gm x 190 lbs., or 95 grams per day. I would like for you to guard against using shark as your sole therapy for treating a recurrence of prostate cancer and strongly recommend that it be used with either a traditional or nontraditional treatment for prostate cancer.

Dr. Lane claims that "it appears that 7 to 8 grams of shark cartilage daily may prevent recurrence" of cancer, particularly if one's lifestyle includes good nutrition and a normal body weight. Shark cartilage can be administered in several ways to achieve rapid absorption. It can be administered orally as pills, rectally as suppositories, or via skin patches that allow the agent to be absorbed directly into the skin. Some physicians believe that when treating advanced stage cancer patients, enzymes and other nutrients are often more effective when given via retention enemas than when administered orally. WARN-

ING: Shark cartilage blocks the body's ability to generate new blood vessels. Therefore, if you have ever suffered a heart attack or recently had major surgery, you should not take shark cartilage.

A colleague in my prostate cancer support group in Brooklyn, New York, who has had a recurrence of prostate cancer is taking shark cartilage as well as another nutrient called sun chlorella which can be purchased at most health food stores. I personally feel that he should have been treated first with combination hormonal therapy to arrest that disease, and then begun taking the two nutrients. However, the best advice I can give you is to listen carefully to your doctor and if necessary, ask for scientific evidence to support his or her recommendation.

As implied previously, a healthy mental attitude is a requirement for combatting a recurrence of prostate cancer. Whenever a patient is experiencing psychological problems, biological changes tend to debilitate him. A healthy body must be sponsored by a healthy mind, or both are doomed. In an effort to help foster a healthy mind, I am recommending the following quality of life activities.

Set Some Quality of Life Goals

Research seems to indicate that those who set reasonable goals for themselves and are committed to attaining them will most likely achieve them. If this is true, then I believe you should carefully set some five- to ten-year goals for yourself, and each year set some short-range objectives to attain these goals. Take a look at some of the long-range goals and short-range objectives I set for myself, even though my radiation oncologist believes my disease has been cured or is at least in remission.

Long-Range Quality of Life Goals:

1. To travel extensively to experience the fun and enjoyment of ten places and people throughout the world by the year 2000.
2. To maintain a proper diet (proper diet means no red meat, no dairy food, and no cake, candy, or cookies), exercise a

minimum of three times per week, participate in at least one psychological healing workshop per year, and get a complete physical examination yearly, by the year 2000.

My short-range quality of life objectives to realize the long-range goals are as follows:

1.1 During the year 1994, visit Colorado and view the Grand Canyon.

2.1 During the year 1994, maintain a calendar and indicate on same whenever I maintain my proper diet; Lucille Roberts three times weekly; get a complete examination of prostate, colon, eyes, and diabetic condition; and attend a workshop on healing of the mind.

Understand Your Thoughts and the Healing Process

The good thing about thoughts is that you have the opportunity to change negative thoughts into positive ones. But, to change your thoughts, you should try to look for the goodness in everything and everybody. However, first look for the goodness in yourself and do not let negative people discourage you. For example, when a person says something negative about you, say to yourself, "John is appearance-oriented. With time, he will learn that it is not appearances that count, but your heart."

Try to love everybody. I know this is extremely difficult. It means that you must know your own weaknesses and how these affect your thoughts, decisions, and actions. Loving everybody does not mean that you have to tell people that you love them, but you must demonstrate that love through your deeds, words, and thoughts. One way to do this is to minimize your negative judgements of people. Whenever I am confronted with negative thoughts about someone, I usually think or reply: I am not God; I cannot judge; I just do not know all the facts.

Positive thoughts will help heal your prostate condition; negative thoughts will debilitate your disease. Believe in yourself. Belief that you will be cured of your disease will enable you to live longer regardless of the stage of your prostate cancer. Do not give up if the last pages of this book are being turned. Only God is reading your book of life and He alone knows when yours will end.

A simple thought can have a significant impact on your mind, body, and emotions. Try this out:

Go into a quiet room of your house. Close the door. Think of a lemon. Imagine cutting it in half. Imagine removing the seeds with the point of a knife. Bring the lemon up to your nose. Smell the lemon. Now, imagine squeezing the juice from the lemon into your mouth. Now, imagine digging your teeth into the center of the lemon. Chew the pulp of the lemon. Feel those little things breaking and popping inside your mouth. (Author unknown)

If you are like most people, your salivary glands respond to the thought of a lemon. Even though you did not actually chew the lemon, your body and mind reacted as though you did. Thoughts have a power over mind, body, and emotions. I remember an incident I read about World War II with the Japanese in which some American troops gave up their lives because they could no longer tolerate the torture administered by the Japanese soldiers. They would actually produce thoughts in their minds to die during the night. And they did. They in effect willed themselves to death. The same thing can happen to you unless you take control over your negative thoughts.

Positive thoughts (joy, life, happiness, fulfillment, achievement) will have a positive impact on your body, such as calm, love, and enthusiasm. On the other hand, negative thoughts (death, resentment, mistrust) will have a negative impact on your body, such as tension, fear, anger, etc. In an effort to control your thoughts, the following are some activities you should engage in. Since your thoughts do impact your healing process, you should begin a daily process of healing yourself psychologically by engaging in several activities so they become habit-forming. Some of these activities are delineated

below; however, for an in-depth study of these activities, see
the references identified in the bibliography.

Visualize Good Health

Carl Simonton, M.D., has for years used the nontraditional
methods for treating cancer patients diagnosed as terminal.
When new patients enter his clinic for an initial consultation
and indicate gloomy remarks about their condition, he looks
them straight in the eye and asks, "When did you decide to
die?" The idea works this way: Imagine whatever is not healthy
about you as the Bad Guys and your own healthy body parts
as the Good Guys. Then, imagine them fighting it out. Of
course, the Good Guys always win.

For example, my prostate cancer was located in two sites
of my prostate. Each time I got a dose of radiation treatment,
I visualized that the linear accelerator (the equipment used to
irradiate my prostate tumor) was a machine gun firing on two
fronts of my prostate to rid me of the disease. The combination
hormonal therapy I received was like planes dropping bombs
on my prostate tumor to downstage and debulk my disease.

Make Affirmative Statements About Good Health

An affirmation is a positive statement to help your healing
process. It is always stated in the present and usually begins
with "I am." Affirmations are designed to make firm positive
statements about yourself. They can be said anywhere, silently
or outloud. The more often you say them, the more real, true,
solid, and firm they become. It really does not matter where
you say them; however, it is better if you look into your eyes
through a mirror.

Create affirmation statements that are related to your condition. Keep them positive and focus on the present, the here
and now. Say, "*I am* beating prostate cancer." Do not say, "*I
want* to beat prostate cancer." The following are some affirmation statements to get you started. Review these and then create
your own.

- "I will not die because I have not fulfilled my purpose yet."
- "I will fight this disease until the end—its end."
- "I will conquer my prostate cancer."
- "I am strong and determined; my disease is weak and powerless."
- "I will destroy my cancerous tumor through thoughts, words, and actions."
- "I am on the side of God; my disease is on the side of the devil. God will prevail in the end."

Heal Through Forgiveness

Forgiveness may be the best healing activity of all. As human beings, we hold so much against ourselves and against others that we cripple ourselves psychologically. As a result, we build up so many emotional illnesses that it prevents us from living a positive and meaningful life. How do we get out of this rut? Through forgiveness. How do we accomplish forgiveness? All you have to do is to use a stem statement and say, "I forgive myself for"_____ or "I forgive_____(another person) for ..." and fill in the blanks.

The following are some forgiveness statements:

- "I forgive myself for fearing prostate cancer."
- "I forgive my doctor for not explaining the options I have for treatment of prostate cancer."

Next, declare judgmental forgiveness statements, as cited in the following statements:

- "I forgive myself for judging myself for _____."
- "I forgive myself for judging my doctor's associate for being responsible for my late cancer diagnosis."

The fact that we did something or someone else did something is not the real problem. The real problem for us begins when we judge what happened as either bad, wrong, improper, harmful, etc. It is our judgment we should really forgive. Our judgment that the action was harmful, etc., is really not what causes our difficulty. If you are going to judge someone or something, do not rely on hunches, guesses, or intuition. Instead, wait until all the information is in, and rely more on facts, hard data, and research. Forgive yourself and everybody. Nothing from the past should pollute your present. Forgiveness is usually a matter of forgiving yourself. I find an effective way to do this is to stay in the present, or as one author wrote, "be here now."

Commit Yourself to Life

Regardless of what you think about your posture regarding life or death, commit yourself fully to life. By commitment I mean committing yourself to living each moment of your life fully, productively, and joyfully. Commit yourself to everything decent and good for you. Make your commitment a here and now reality rather than some abstract dream. Do not let any negatives seep into your thoughts. Do not say, "I do not know how to live a long, healthy and happy life, therefore, I cannot commit myself. As one author said, ""Commit yourself first, then set out on a cause to discover how to do it." This activity can be summed up in a quote, "The willingness to do creates the ability to do." Be committed to living your life regardless of the condition of your prostate cancer, and the ability, techniques, methods, and activities to do this will emerge.

You Can Have Anything But Not Everything You Want

Regardless of how powerful we are as human beings, there are some significant limitations we all share. For example: 1) we can only be in one place at one time; 2) we have only twenty-four hours in each day; 3) we all must die some time; and 4) we all experience pain and happiness during the course of living.

To obtain what you want will require at least ten steps. If you keep in mind that you cannot have everything you want, the following are ways in which you can get anything you want.

1. Focus all your energy on what you want. Become a maniac for it.
2. Visualize and imagine yourself doing and getting whatever you want.
3. Become obsessed with getting it and having it. For example, although a colleague in one of my prostate cancer support groups was scheduled to undergo a radical prostatectomy, he continued attending prostate cancer support groups, visiting numerous hospitals, and interacting with hospitals. After several months, he finally settled on cryosurgery.
4. Know exactly what you want. Draw a picture of your current prostate gland condition and then next to it draw how it should look when it is cured of the disease.
5. Become driven by what you want.
6. Oppose everything preventing you from getting what you want.
7. Pretend frequently throughout your daily life that you already have what you want.
8. Be grateful for what you already have.
9. Have faith with involvement. Know that you can have what you want if you are involved with whatever you need to do to obtain it.
10. Do whatever is required to get what you want. Work hard at it until you get it.

If your disease has recurred and if only one person has been cured of the disease with combination hormonal therapy, this could be the blueprint for you to recover. As long as one person survives prostate cancer that has metastasized, then you can become number two. And if no one has survived a Stage D3 prostate cancer condition, you could be number one. The struggle after a recurrence of prostate cancer is not between the habit of negative thinking and the positive focus required to heal your body of prostate cancer; the struggle is between remaining here in your present body on this earth or going to another place that many people have described as far greater than where we are.

Take Good Care of Yourself

There are many common sense guidelines for taking care of yourself to enhance your healing process. Most good doctors take for granted that you are already doing these things. Maybe you are; maybe you are not. I have only slightly discussed the need to integrate physical healing with psychological healing. I think this is a good place to begin to close this section; that is, by listing those guidelines you should already be committed to in your healing process.

- Get sufficient rest. While there is no set formula, I would recommend eight hours each night.

- Take vitamins. Check with your health care practitioner to determine which ones are vital for your recovery. Some are mentioned in this chapter.

- Eat sensibly. According to this book, you can indulge yourself in a normal diet as advocated by the National Cancer Institute in Chapter Nine or place yourself on a macrobiotic diet.

- Maintain a reasonable weight. Determine what is the average weight for you according to your height and maintain it plus or minus ten pounds.

- Maintain a three-day per week exercise program. I am on a Nautilus program whereby the equipment dictates the routine exercise that I put by body through.

- Get massages. Recently, a company in New York called the Great Massage established a massage program in which both men and women can attend and pay a fee of less than eight dollars to get an eight-minute back massage. If your community has such a program, make good use of it frequently. Massage releases tension, frees energy, releases physical blocks, and makes you feel good.

- Take hot baths. Take time out of your busy life and take a hot bath to relax. Notice, I did not say shower. Soaking in the tub for a few minutes relaxes the body and soothes the mind.

Have You Fulfilled Your Purpose in Life?

I believe that God has put man and woman on earth to achieve a given purpose. The problem is that most people do not know or have not thought about their purpose in life. Mary Wollstonecraft Shelley said, "Nothing contributes so much to tranquilize the mind as a steady purpose—a point on which the soul may fix its intellectual eye."

A purpose is a simple statement about why you are here and what you are here to do. For example, my purpose in life is to improve the quality of life of people through education. My creation of my purpose took years of learning, teaching, and experiencing. It did not happen overnight. It took time for me to discover it. As I said before, some people never realize they have a purpose in life. As a result, they live from day to day with no guidance and no direction. It was Benjamin Disraeli who said, "The secret of success is constancy to purpose."

A purpose in life gives you meaning and hope for the future. When you have a purpose, your energy will flow to fulfill that purpose. The tension in your body will diminish; as a result, you find meaning and will become more active, vehement, alive, and healthy. Since my purpose is endless, I believe that I must continually strive to attain it, one life at a time.

We All Must Die; Prepare for it Now!

Previously, I have attempted to introduce you to how to integrate your physical healing with your dietary and psychological healing. I believe it is also appropriate to suggest how to prepare yourself for death. Here are some suggestions that you should keep conscious of and use when you think they are appropriate.

Suggestion 1: Take care of business, as indicated in Chapter Nine. Basically, this means get all of your debts in order and do whatever you can so you do not impose them on your family. It is unfair for you to burden your loved ones with your personal debts when they were not involved in creating them. Keep a diary of everything you have done to prepare for the last chapter of life so your family will know what needs to be done after your death. Destroy everything you do not want anyone to see or that will hurt them. Give a gift as a memento to all those you feel enhanced the quality of your life.

Suggestion 2: Make certain all appropriate papers are in order. These include your last will and testament, your living will, a power of attorney for your wife, a health care proxy, as well as your insurance policies and other important documents.

Suggestion 3: Commit to telling your relatives and friends that you love them whenever the occasion arises and thank them for enhancing the quality of your life.

Suggestion 4: Spend time by yourself. Reflect on what you have accomplished in life. Forgive yourself for not accomplishing more, because we usually feel that we could have done more or could have had a better relationship with a relative, friend, or loved one. Think of the good times you had in your life. Although I may not depart tomorrow, I continually think of the wonderful moments of my life, such as when my mother came to my college graduation and the pinning of my officer's bars; the day my oldest son, who was four years old at the time, hugged both my legs and cried because he was delighted that I bought him his first bicycle; the wonderful feeling I felt for my wife when she came home from delivering our first-born child; the excitement I felt over the birth of our first grandchild, Kelsey; the time we gave our daughter a brand new automobile and tears of joy cascaded down her cheeks; and the day I received a fellowship from Harvard University. Each one of these experiences bring joy and happiness to me each and every time I think of them.

Suggestion 5: I find it very convenient to pray to almighty God when I am riding in my car. Sometimes I apologize for any sins I have committed. I constantly think about what I will say to God when I get to the other side of the tunnel when He questions me as to what I have done with my life. I feel confident that He will be delighted.

Suggestion 6: Cry if you want to. Let out all of your grief. I often cry when I hear a familiar tune that triggers the memory of the loss of my mother, brothers, sister, other relatives, or friends. I cry because I miss them dearly and did not realize how much I would miss them. Sometimes I cry because of a sorrowful event in a movie or when I read a book. Other times, I cry because of something good that has happened to somebody. I cry because I want to share my emotions with someone. It is perfectly all right for you to cry, too.

Suggestion 7: Make a list of things you want to see and do as indicated when I asked you to consider preparing a list of quality life goals and objectives to be attained by you. These goals and objectives are basically things you want to see and do before making your departure. My list includes the following:

1. Go to Grand Canyon.
2. Take a trip to Argentina.
3. Attend an Olympic event.
4. Go to La Scala in Italy.
5. Appear on radio or television to deliver a message about prostate cancer.
6. Go to visit the Lady of Fatima.
7. Visit Africa.
8. See more of my relatives.
9. Visit five of the best vacation spots in the world.
10. Heal someone. Although I may not be able to put forth my hands and heal someone, perhaps this book will do the job.

Suggestion 8: Enjoy yourself and others. Think of the people you want to associate with who will make you happy. Take the opportunity to be with them. I really enjoy being with my grandchild and I take every opportunity to be with her. I want very badly for her to come to know her grandfather.

Suggestion 9: Enjoy each remaining moment of your life. Be here now. Do not concentrate on the past or the future. The here and now is where you will find happiness. You may have only a few more pages of your life; make the most of them now.

Suggestion 10: When it is time to go, let go. Do what you think is necessary to let go without lingering. It may mean preparing a living will or making arrangements for your funeral. It may mean going off somewhere to make your departure.

As you may have noticed, many of these items sound more like suggestions for living than for dying. That is because the best way to prepare yourself for death is to live each and every moment as if it is the last day of your life. When your book of life has been closed, it is perhaps because it is the beginning of another life, in another person, in another time.

If you have a recurrence of prostate cancer, do not give up. This should make you more determined to continue your struggle with the disease. Just think, if you can conquer this disease with additional physical, dietary, and psychological healings, you will be a prime example for the rest of the men in the world to emulate. You will become a champion over prostate cancer, just like Ney, whom I discussed earlier in this book. Even if you are not able to overcome the recurrence of prostate cancer, just the mere fact that you tried and enhanced the quality of your life in the process is worth the effort. God be with you.

Glossary

Abdomen: The part of the body located below the ribs and above the pelvic bone.

Adjuvant therapy: A treatment method used in addition to the primary therapy. Radiation therapy is often used as an adjuvant to surgery.

Adrenal glands: Two glands located above the kidneys (one above each kidney). They produce several kinds of hormones, including a small amount of sex hormones.

Androgens: Male sex hormones produced by the testicles and, in small amounts, by the adrenal glands.

Anesthesia: Loss of feeling or sensation resulting from the use of certain drugs or gases.

Angiogenesis: The formation of new blood vessels.

Antiangiogenesis: Preventing the development of new blood vessels.

Anus: The opening at the lower end of the rectum through which solid waste is eliminated.

Benign: A nonmalignant or noncancerous condition.

Benign Prostatic Hyperplasia/Benign Prostatic Hypertrophy (BPH):   A noncancerous, yet serious condition of the prostate; generally, an enlargement of the gland, causing obstruction of urination, which can result in secondary complications.

Bilateral Orchiectomy: Surgical removal of the testicles to halt production of testosterone.

Biopsy: The procedure to obtain tissue, which is then examined by a pathologist using a microscope to distinguish between cancerous and noncancerous conditions; for prostate cancer this may be a needle biopsy, or transurectal resection of the prostate (TUR/P).

Bladder: The hollow organ that stores urine.

Blood chemistry: Analysis of multiple components in the serum (blood), including tests to evaluate function of the liver and kidneys, minerals, cholesterol, etc.; important especially because abnormal values can indicate spread of cancer, or side effects of treatment(s).

Blood count: Analysis, primarily of red blood cells (which help transport oxygen in the body), white blood cells (which protect against infection), and platelets (necessary for clotting of blood); abnormal values can indicate cancerous involvement of the bone marrow, or side effects of the treatment(s).

Brachytherapy: Treatment with radioactive sources placed into or very near the tumor in the affected area; includes surface application, body cavity application, and placement into the tissue. Sometimes this term is used interchangeably with "internal radiation therapy."

CT scan (Computerized Tomography):   A computer-assisted type of X-ray, allowing detailed visualization of the body; particularly useful in evaluating soft-tissue organs.

Cancer: A general term for more than 100 diseases in which abnormal cells multiply without control. Cancer cells can spread through the bloodstream and lymphatic system to the other parts of the body.

Castration: Elimination of testicular function, either by surgical removal of the testes (surgical castration), or by administration of an LHRH analog (a class of drugs designed to inhibit testicular function).

Carcinoma: Cancer that begins in the lining or covering of an organ.

Catheterization: Inserting a catheter through the urethra into the bladder.

Chemotherapy: Treatment with anticancer drugs.

Clinical trials: Studies conducted with patients, usually to evaluate a promising new drug or treatment. Each study is designed to answer scientific questions and find better ways to treat patients.

Cobalt 60:   A radioactive substance used as a radiation source to treat cancer.

Cystoscope: A lighted instrument used to look at the inside of the bladder.

Diagnosis: Evaluation of symptoms and/or tests leading to the verification of the existence of an abnormal condition.

Diploid: Slow-growing prostate cancer cells.

Ejaculation: The release of semen through the penis during orgasm.

Estrogen: A female sex hormone.

External radiation therapy: Treatment with high energy radiation given from a source located outside the body.

Flow Cytometry: The process by which graphs or histograms are plotted based on the DNA content of the cancerous tissue cells.

Foley Catheter: In terms of men, a foley catheter is a tube that is inserted through the tip of the penis into the urethra until it enters the bladder.

Hormone: A chemical substance that is formed in one part of the body, travels through the blood, and affects the function of cells elsewhere in the body.

Hormone therapy: Treatment that prevents cancer cells from getting the hormones they need to grow. Hormone therapy for prostate cancer keeps the cancer cells from getting male hormones. Treatment may involve removing the testicles or giving female hormones or other drugs to prevent the production of male hormones or to block their effect on cancer cells.

Hyperthermia: Using heat produced by microwave radiation to treat prostate cancer.

Implant: A small container of radioactive material placed in or near a cancer.

Impotence: Partial or complete loss of erection, which may be associated with a loss of libido; may be a result of injury secondary to radiation therapy or surgical resection of the prostate, which may or may not be permanent, or may be a result of hormone deprivation therapy.

Incision: A cut made during surgery.

Incontinence: Partial or complete loss of urine control; may be a result of injury secondary to radiation therapy or surgical resection of the prostate.

Internal radiation: A type of therapy in which a radioactive substance is implanted into or close to the area needing treatment.

Interstitial implant: A radioactive source placed directly into the tissue (not in a body cavity).

Intravenous pyelogram: X-rays of the kidneys, ureters, and bladder taken after a dye is injected into a vein. Also called IVP.

Linear accelerator: A machine that creates high energy radiation to treat cancers using electricity to form a stream of fast moving subatomic particles.

Local therapy: Treatment that affects a tumor and tissue near it.

Luteinizing hormone-releasing hormone: A hormone that controls sex hormones in men and women. Also called LHRH.

Luteinizing hormone-releasing hormone (LHRH) agonist:
A substance that closely resembles LHRH, which controls the production of sex hormones. However, LHRH agonists affect the body differently than does LHRH. LHRH agonists keep the testicles from producing hormones.

Lymph: The almost colorless fluid that travels through the lymphatic system and carries cells that help fight infection.

Lymph nodes: Small, bean-shaped organs located along the channels of the lymphatic system. The lymph nodes store special cells that can trap bacteria or cancer cells traveling through the body in lymph nodes. Also called lymph glands.

Lymphadenectomy: The surgical removal of one or more lymph nodes for purposes of microscopic examination; may be performed as an "open pelvic lymphadenectomy" as the initial approach during radical prostatectomy, or a separate procedure prior to radical prostatectomy by means of small incision(s) into the pelvic cavity ("laparoscopic lymphadenectomy").

Lymphatic system: The tissues and organs that produce, store, and carry cells that fight infection and disease. This system includes the bone marrow, spleen, thymus, lymph nodes, and channels that carry lymph.

MRI (Magnetic Resonance Imaging) scan: A sophisticated use of an electromagnet and sound waves to create a detailed X-ray type image by measurement of signal intensity of a particular body part or region; in general, this may be the most effective means of detecting whether the tumor has penetrated through the capsule of the prostate gland and/or invaded the seminal vesicle(s), and can be used to evaluate whether pelvic lymph nodes are enlarged.

Malignant: Cancerous; can spread to other parts of the body.

Metastasis: (plural is metastases):   Spread or transfer of a malignant tumor to another part of the body not directly connected to the original tumor location; all malignant (cancerous) tumors have the potential to metastasize (spread), while benign conditions do not.

Moderately Differentiated: A classification of prostate cancer in which the cells are beginning to lose their shape and is graded between 5 and 8.

Oncologist: A doctor who specializes in treating cancer. Some oncologists specialize in a particular type of cancer treatment. For example, a radiation oncologist treats cancer with radiation.

Orchiectomy: Surgery to remove the testicles.

Palliative therapy: A treatment that may relieve symptoms without curing the disease.

Pathologist: A doctor who identifies disease by studying cells and tissues under a microscope.

Pelvic: Referring to the area of the body located at below the waist and surrounded by the hip and pubic bones.

Perineal prostatectomy: Surgery to remove the prostate through an incision made between the scrotum and the anus.

Poorly Differentiated: A late classification of prostate cancer in which there is no definite shape of the cells and is graded between 9 and 10.

Primary: A term that refers to the organ, gland, etc., where the cancer begins, from which it may then spread (for example, "primary" prostate cancer which may "metastasize" to the bone).

Prognosis: The probable outcome or course of a disease; the chance of recovery.

Progression: A term used to describe continued growth of the cancer, or recurrence of cancer after a previous response to treatment.

Prostate: A male sex gland; it produces a fluid that forms part of semen.

Prostate acid phosphatase: An enzyme produced by the prostate that is elevated in some patients with prostate cancer.

Prostate-specific antigen: A protein whose level in the blood goes up in some men who have prostate cancer or benign prostatic hyperplasia. Also called PSA.

Prostate Specific Antigen (PSA) Assay: A blood test for the measurement of a substance produced by prostate gland cells; used both for screening (an elevation of the PSA indicates an abnormal condition of the prostate gland, either benign or malignant, requiring further investigation for diagnosis), and to monitor the progress of a patient undergoing treatment and/or after surgery or radiation therapy; it is the most sensitive "marker" of prostate cancer that is currently available.

Prostatectomy: An operation to remove part or all of the prostate.

Prostate acid phosphatase: An enzyme produced by the prostate. Its level in the blood goes up in some men who have prostate cancer. Also called PAP.

Prostatic Acid Phosphatase (PAP) Assay: A blood test to measure a substance most notably (not exclusively) produced by prostate gland cells; also useful as a "marker" because the PAP is typically elevated if there is metastasis.

Rad: Short form for "radiation absorbed dose;" a measurement of the amount of radiation absorbed by tissues (100 rad = 1 gray).

Radiation: Energy carried by waves or a stream of particles.

Radiation therapy: Treatment with high energy rays from X-rays or other sources to damage cancer cells. The radiation may come from a machine (external radiation therapy) or from radioactive materials placed inside the body as close as possible to the cancer (internal radiation therapy).

Radiaton Oncologist: A physician with special training in reading diagnostic X-rays and performing specialized X-ray procedures

Radiation physicist: A person trained to ensure that the radiation machine delivers the right amount of radiation to the treatment site.

Radical prostatectomy: Surgery to remove the entire prostate. The two types of radical prostatectomy are retropubic prostatectomy and perineal prostatectomy.

Radiotherapy: See radiation therapy.

Rectal exam: A procedure in which a doctor inserts a gloved, lubricated finger into the rectum and feels the prostate through the wall of the rectum to check the prostate for hard or lumpy areas.

Refractory: A term used most commonly to describe the situation when the disease is no longer controlled by current therapy; similar to "progression."

Remission: Disappearance of the signs and symptoms of cancer. When this happens, the disease is said to be "in remission." Remission can be temporary or permanent.

Response: A decrease in the extent of disease as evidenced by reduction or disappearance of visible tumor and/or markers, which may be complete or partial; because untreated cancers are generally progressive, stability (no change) of disease is sometimes considered to be a positive response to treatment.

Retropubic prostatectomy: Surgical removal of the prostate through an incision in the abdomen.

Scrotum: The external pouch of skin that contains the testicles.

Semen: The fluid that is released through the penis during orgasm. Semen is made up of sperm from the testicles and fluid from the prostate and other sex glands.

Simulation: A process involving special X-ray pictures that are used to plan radiation treatment so the areas to be treated are precisely located and marked for treatment.

Stage: A categorical assessment of the degree to which a cancer has grown at the time of initial diagnosis or at a point of reevaluation; a very simple implication is that the more advanced the stage of disease may be, there is greater likelihood that the disease represents a potentially fatal illness.

Staging: The actual process of categorically assessing the extent of prostate cancer.

TRUS-P (Transrectal Ultrasound of the Prostate):   A test using soundwave echoes to create an image of an organ or gland to visually inspect for abnormal conditions; helpful in assessing the prostate gland for enlargement, nodules, and penetration of the tumor through the capsule of the gland and/or invasion of the seminal vesicle(s); extremely useful for guidance of needle biopsies of the prostate gland.

TUR/P (Transurectal Resection of the Prostate): A surgical procedure by which small portions of the prostate gland are removed through incision of the inside of the urethra (through the penis); a TUR/P is often performed to relieve obstruction of urine flow because of compression of urethra due to enlargement of the prostate; many times unsuspected cancer is discovered in the resected specimen when this procedure is done for presumed benign enlargement of the prostate gland.

Testicles: The two egg-shaped glands that produce sperm and male hormones.

Testosterone: A male sex hormone.

Transurethral resection: The use of a special instrument inserted through the penis to remove a small prostate tumor. This procedure can also be accomplished by laser.

Tumor: An abnormal mass of tissue. Tumors are either benign or malignant.

Ultrasound: A technique that uses sound waves that cannot be heard by humans to produce pictures of areas inside the body. The pictures are created by a computer that analyzes the echoes produced by the waves as they bounce off tissues.

Ureter: The tube that carries urine from each kidney to the bladder.

Urethra: The tube that carries urine or semen to the outside of the body.

Urologist: A doctor who specializes in diseases of the urinary organs in females and the urinary and sex organs in males.

Well-differentiated: An early classification of prostate cancer in which the cells have definite shape and is graded between 1 and 4.

X-ray: High energy radiation that can be used at low levels to diagnose disease or at high levels to treat cancer.

References

CHAPTER 1: *What I Learned and What You Should Know About Prostate Cancer*

1. Das, Sakti, and David E. Crawford, Eds. *Cancer of the Prostate.* New York, NY: Marcel Dekker, Inc., 1993, pp. 39-94. A technical, but very helpful source for learning more about prostate cancer.

2. *Cancer Communication Prostate Cancer Report.* Grand Rapids, MI: PAACT, Inc., 1992, pp. 14-24.

3. *Cancer Communication Prostate Cancer Report.* Grand Rapids, MI: PAACT, Inc., 1992, pp. 1-64.

   This source proved to be very comprehensive in that it facilitated my grasp of the subject.

CHAPTER 2: *Understanding Your Choices of Treatment for Prostate Cancer*

1. Information on I-125 seed implantation was obtained from *Another Therapeutic Approach to Prostate Cancer: Radioactive Seed Implantation.* Arlington Heights, IL: Medi-Physics, Inc., 1992, pp. 3-8.

CHAPTER 3: *Some Questionable Practices I Discovered in the Diagnosis and Treatment of Prostate Cancer*

I arrived at the questionable practices cited through reading numerous books and articles, some of which are cited in the bibliography. My reasons are based on some of the current research as well as my opinions, which may be in conflict with members of the medical profession.

CHAPTER 4: *What I Did to Gain Support and Acquire Knowledge About My Condition*

1. The information about US TOO was obtained from the April/May 1993 edition of the *US TOO* newsletter.

2. The information on PAACT was obtained from several editions of the organization's newsletters, *Cancer Communication*, 1990 to 1993.

CHAPTER 5: *How to Select and Communicate With Your Doctor*

1. Lobanov, Silvia. *Keys to Choosing a Doctor*. Hauppauge, NY: Barron's Educational Services, Inc., 1991, pp. 72-74.

   Some of the information pertaining to selecting a doctor came from this source.

2. My other source of information in writing the contents of this chapter came from a visit to one of US TOO's prostate cancer support groups at the Sloan Memorial-Kettering Cancer Center in New York.

CHAPTER 6: *Thank God for Flutamide*

1. *Cancer Communication Prostate Cancer Report*. Grand Rapids, MI: PAACT, Inc., 1992, pp. 19-24.

I could not have written this chapter had it not been for the research cited in this book. Although this book is designed for medical students, I found it helpful for citing some of the research on this topic.

2. Das, Sakti, and David E. Crawford, Eds. *Cancer of the Prostate.* New York, NY: Marcel Dekker, Inc., 1993, pp. 333-368.

    This book is an excellent source for learning about what you can expect at each step of radical prostatectomy. Permission was granted for reprinting the quotes cited in the text.

CHAPTER 7: *What You Should Know Before, During, and After Your Prostate Cancer Treatment*

1. Rous, Stephen N. *The Prostate Book.* Yonkers, NY: Consumer Reports Books, 1992, pp. 162-177; 180-204.

2. Information on I-125 seed implantation was obtained from *Another Therapeutic Approach to Prostate Cancer: Radioactive Seed Implantation.* Arlington Heights, IL: Medi-Physics, Inc., 1992, pp. 3-8.

3. U.S. Department of Health and Human Services. *Radiation Therapy and You,* 1990.

    This guide was helpful to me in the section on radiation therapy. Obviously, my own experience in external beam radiation also proved to be helpful.

CHAPTER 8: *Questions and Answers About Prostate Cancer*

Similar to Chapter 3, the questions and answers cited in this chapter are based on my reading, research, and thoughts and may be in conflict with members of the medical profession.

1. Hamand, Jeremy. *Prostate Problems*. London, England: Thorsons Self-Help Series, 1991, p. 130.

The information on the incidence of prostate cancer worldwide was obtained from this publication.

CHAPTER 9: *What You and Your Partner May Want to Know About the Impact of Prostate Cancer*

Three books which were very useful for me to write Chapter Nine are as follows:

1. Gomella, Leonard G., and John J. Fried. *Recovering From Prostate Cancer*. New York, NY: Harper Paperbacks, 1993, pp. 116-158.

2. Hamand, Jeremy. *Prostate Problems*. London, England: Thorsons Self-Help Series, 1991, pp. 101-144.

3. Morganstern, Steven, and Allen Abrahams. *The Prostate Sourcebook*. Los Angeles, CA: Lowell House, 1993, pp. 109-142.

CHAPTER 10: *What You Should Do If You Have a Recurrence of Prostate Cancer*

1. Borysenko, John. *Minding the Body, Mending the Mind*. Bantam Books, New York, NY: 1988, pp. 9-28; 89-110; 137-158.

When my daughter found out I was closing my book by recommending healing the body using psychological healing, she referred me to this book, which I found to be extremely helpful in preparing the content of this chapter.

2. Kushi, Michio. *The Cancer Prevention Diet*. New York, NY: St. Martin's Press, 1983, pp. 264-277.

I obtained the substance of the research regarding prostate cancer from this source as well as what foods are appropriate for preventing and healing the body with prostate cancer.

3. The source I used to discuss the use of shark cartilage to prevent or treat prostate cancer came from Dr. I. William Lane's book entitled *Sharks Don't Get Cancer: How Shark Cartilage Could Save Your Life*. Garden City Park, NY: Avery Publishing Group, Inc., 1992.

4. Roger, John, and Peter McWilliams. *You Can't Afford the Luxury of a Negative Thought*. Los Angeles, CA: Prelude Press, 1991, pp. 45-46; 157-160; 213-218; 303-304; 499-504; 557-562; 579-582.

I used certain topics cited in this book to elaborate on the psychological aspects of healing. Many of the psychological healing activities cited in this source proved invaluable to me as I related them to prostate cancer patients.

Bibliography

Borysenko, Joan. *Minding the Body, Mending the Mind.* New York, NY: Bantam Books, 1988.

Chaitow, Leon. *Prostate Troubles.* London, England: Thorsons Self-Help Series, 1988.

Chopra, Deepak. *Quantum Healing.* New York, NY: Bantam Books, 1989.

Cunningham, Chet. *The Prostate Problem: The Guide to What Every Man Over 40 Needs to Know and Why!* New York, NY: Pinnacle Books, 1990.

Das, Sakti, and E. David Crawford, Eds. *Cancer of the Prostate.* New York, NY: Marcel Dekker, Inc., 1993.

Fine, Judith. *Afraid to Ask: A Book for Families to Share About Cancer.* New York, NY: Lothrop, Lee, and Shephard, 1986.

Fitzpatrick, John M., and Robert J. Krane, Eds. *The Prostate.* New York, NY: Churchill Livingstone, 1989.

Garrison, Judith Garrett, and Scott Shepherd. *Cancer and Hope.* Minneapolis, MN: CompCare Publishers, 1991.

Gomella, Leonard G., M.D., and John J. Fried. *Recovering From Prostate Cancer: A Doctor's Guide for Patients and Their Loved Ones.* New York, NY: HarperCollins Publishers, 1993.

Graham, Jory. *In the Company of Others: Understanding the Human Needs of Cancer Patients.* New York, NY: Harcourt Brace Jovanovich, 1982.

Harpham, Wendy Schlessel, M.D. *Diagnosis Cancer: Your Guide Through the First Few Months.* New York, NY: W.W. Norton and Co., 1992.

Hay, Louise L. *You Can Heal Your Life.* Carson, CA: Hay House, Inc., 1993.

Kushi, Michio. *The Cancer Prevention Diet.* New York, NY: St. Martin's Press, 1983.

Lane, I. William. *Sharks Don't Get Cancer.* Garden City Park, NY: Avery Publishing Group, Inc., 1993.

Lobanov, Igor, and Silvia Valdivieso-Lobanov. *Keys to Choosing a Doctor.* Hauppauge, NY: Barron's Educational Series, Inc., 1991.

Locke, Steven, and Douglas Colligan. *The Healer Within: The New Medicine of Mind and Body.* New York, NY: E.P. Dutton, 1986.

Morganstern, Steven, M.D., and Allen Abrahams, Ph.D. *The Prostate Sourcebook.* Chicago, IL: Lowell House, 1993.

Morva, Marion, and Eve Potts. *Choices: Realistic Alternatives in Cancer Treatment.* New York, NY: Avon Books, 1987.

Ney, Lloyd J. *Prostate Cancer Report.* Grand Rapids, MI: PAACT, Inc., 1992.

Roger, John, and Peter McWilliams. *You Can't Afford the Luxury of a Negative Thought.* Los Angeles, CA: Prelude Press, 1991.

Rous, Stephen N. *The Prostate Book.* Yonkers, NY: Consumer Report Books, 1992.

Shook, Robert. *Survivors Living With Cancer: Portraits of Twelve Inspiring People.* New York, NY: Harper and Row, 1983.

Weil, Andrew. *Health and Healing: Understanding Conventional and Alternative Medicine.* Boston, MA: Houghton Mifflin, 1983.

Weisman, Avery D. *Coping With Cancer.* New York, NY: McGraw-Hill, 1979.

INDEX